24
ways
to
move
more

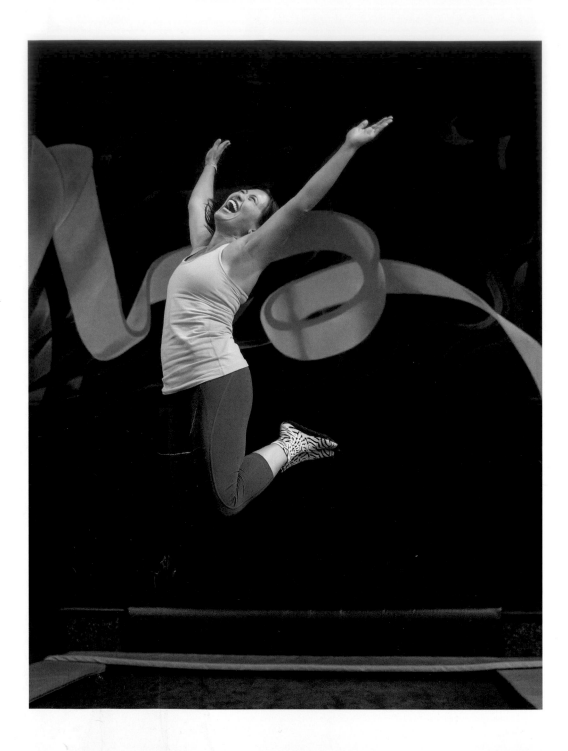

24
ways
to
move
more

Monthly Inspiration for Health & Movement

NICOLE TSONG

Photography by ERIKA SCHULTZ

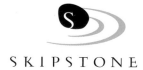

SKIPSTONE

To the movers of the world

Copyright © 2020 by Nicole Tsong
Photography © by Erika Schultz
All rights reserved. No part of this book may be reproduced or utilized in any form, or by any electronic, mechanical, or other means, without the prior written permission of the publisher.

Published by Skipstone, an imprint of Mountaineers Books—an independent, nonprofit publisher

Skipstone and its colophon are registered trademarks of The Mountaineers organization.
Printed in China
23 22 21 20   1 2 3 4 5

Copyeditor: Ali Shaw, Indigo: Editing, Design, and More
Design: Kate Basart/Union Pageworks
Cover photographs by Erika Schultz
All photographs by Erika Shultz except as follows: page 15 by Mountaineers Books; page 18 © Blazej Lyjak/Deposit Photos; page 117 © Michelangelo Oprandi/DepositPhotos; page 135 by Bill Thorness

Library of Congress Cataloging-in-Publication Data is on file for this title at https://lccn.loc.gov/2020004709.

Printed on FSC®-certified materials

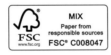

ISBN (paperback): 978-1-68051-274-8
ISBN (ebook): 978-1-68051-275-5

Skipstone books may be purchased for corporate, educational, or other promotional sales, and our authors are available for a wide range of events. For information on special discounts or booking an author, contact our customer service at 800.553.4453 or mbooks@mountaineersbooks.org.

Skipstone
1001 SW Klickitat Way
Suite 201
Seattle, Washington 98134
206.223.6303
www.skipstonebooks.org
www.mountaineersbooks.org

LIVE LIFE. MAKE RIPPLES.

contents

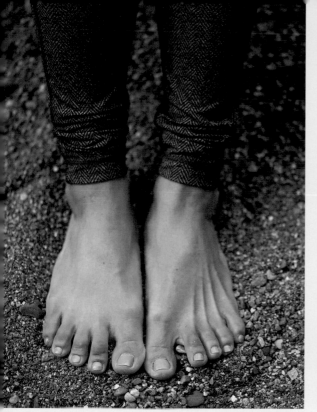
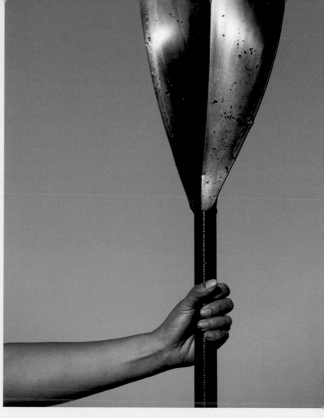

my
movement
journey

I couldn't stop grinning, my hair plastered to my head. I was breathing hard, and I didn't care. I shrieked with laughter as friends bounced me off-balance on a giant blue-and-yellow inflatable tube. I jumped off a tall platform onto a huge inflated landing pad.

Splashing around in a lake on inflatable toys, watching my friend Kristen scream as she flew over the water on a rope swing, cooling off from the intense heat in Texas hill country, I had never felt so strong, so trusting of my body, so happy it could play so hard. Not my adult self, anyway.

I knew, technically, that my strength was above average. For the previous six years, my body had endured long yoga practices several times a week. My legs no longer shook in an extended warrior hold, and I'd made progress on holding a handstand without a wall. For two years, I had taught the sweaty yoga I loved, encouraging my students in a high runner's lunge or when they attempted a new arm balance. I took teacher trainings where practices sometimes lasted five hours, sweat dripping off my nose onto my mat in downward-facing dog.

Even so, I didn't feel like a real mover. Sure, I did yoga four days a week. I felt stronger on hikes than I ever had. But I didn't think of myself as a physical person, surely not an athlete.

But that day, playing at the lake, something inside me clicked. Moving my body in ways outside my norm didn't feel overwhelming or hard. I laughed when other people bounced me off-balance. I raced around like a kid, convinced I could do anything on the inflatable toys scattered across the lake. I was gleeful jumping into the water.

I felt exhilarated—while moving my body.

The experience etched itself into my memory. A couple of years passed before the notion that moving my body was an instant pathway to feeling happy and joyful cemented itself—when I knew in my bones that my body was not only strong and capable but also that moving it was an essential ingredient to feeling good on a daily basis.

Now, I center my life around this fact: moving my body makes me happy.

If you had told me at age 16, 25, or even 30 that I would love moving so much that it would be a mandatory part of daily life, that I would write a weekly fitness column for *The Seattle Times* for six years and then turn it into a book dedicated to getting you to bust a move on the dance floor or lace up a pair of roller skates, you may as well have told me I was going to be an A-list movie star.

But that's exactly what happened. The fitness part, not the movie star part.

A WOBBLY BEGINNING

Perhaps the memory of Dorothy Hamill and her 1976 Olympic gold medal lingered into the early 1980s, so it made sense to my mom that her two girls should learn to fly across the ice. Michelle Kwan was only a toddler then, years away from her Olympic medals. Credit to my mom for being at the forefront of the trend of Asian-American figure skaters.

At age five, the only reason I stepped out onto the slippery ice was to be like my older sister, Ingrid. I would do anything to keep

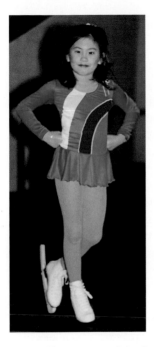

up with her; I even pretended I wanted to ice skate. I didn't like falling on the hard ice, so I skated carefully, going slowly as I stepped one foot over the other doing crossovers in the little rink where I learned to skate forward and backward and to perfect T-stops.

A few years later, my radio alarm clock went off twice a week in the morning darkness, startling me out of sleep. I hit snooze until my mom opened my door and snapped, "Nicole, you up?" I rolled out of bed and stumbled to the bathroom, grumpy that I had to be up so early to practice.

I donned a teal-green zip-up jacket with matching short skirt, shiny tan tights, and scuffed white skates for private lessons with my coach, Yvonne. Yvonne's feathered, grayed-out blonde hair looked almost white. She was taller than me, though not by much, and wore a long blue coat with a fluffy white lining to keep herself warm on the ice. She had kind blue eyes and a maternal quality.

Figure skaters showed up early at the ice arena's parking circle, dropped off one by one, walking over a concrete bridge that crossed a tiny creek. When I opened the doors, the biting-cold smell of ice and dank carpet in the lobby hit my nose. I dropped my heavy duffel bag underneath the carpeted brown benches in the lobby and stuffed my toes into my tight boots, which hurt my feet every time I wore them. I carried clear nail polish in my ice skating bag in case I got a run in my tights.

Once on the ice, shivering, I skated in circles to warm up. Skating fast was the best part of practice. I felt free zooming around the ice. I didn't have to think; muscle memory took over. I went to the same patch of ice every time, spinning on one foot and learning to waltz jump, skating forward on one foot and landing backward on another. I watched older girls throw themselves into difficult double loops or lutzes, stumbling or falling out of the jump and trying again.

One day, when I was eight, I skated up to Yvonne at the hockey bench where we met for my private lessons. Yvonne looked over the top of her glasses, assessing me.

"Nicole, I think it's time for you to compete," she said.

My heart fluttered in my chest. Ingrid was already competing. I envied the confidence of older skaters, heads held high as they danced around the ice in shiny, colorful dresses with shimmery sequins for competitions and the annual ice show. But I didn't want to compete, not really. Skate alone in front of an audience, with people watching me? I squirmed inside.

"Okay," I answered, obedient to my coach.

Yvonne wanted me to compete in freestyle solo and also in compulsory skills, showcasing technique. She asked if I also wanted to do interpretive figure skating, a free-form event where skaters are given an unknown song and don't have a routine.

"No," I said. I had some limits back then.

Yvonne didn't push. She shuffled through her tapes.

"First, we have to figure out a song. Then we can create a program," she said. "Do you want fast music or slow?"

Fast meant I would have to skate faster and jump higher. Fast would push me. Fast sounded terrifying.

"Slow," I answered.

She chose "Rainbow Connection" from *The Muppet Movie*. I practiced my routine until I could do it without thinking, the jumps and the spins ingrained, timed to match every swell of Kermit's voice.

At my first competition, I thought I might throw up waiting for my name to be called. I stood, shaking, at the side of rink. Yvonne rubbed my arms as I waited. Once I was on the ice, posing in my starting position in a new blue dress adorned with white and maroon sequins, the familiar strains of the song floated toward me. I moved, extending my arms side to side and following the program stamped into my muscles.

It took me years to understand the gift of my early years of ice skating and competition. I was much older before I appreciated how it cultivated balance and strength, how I learned discipline from the early morning practices, how the challenge of performing in front of people was my first step to rising into something bigger than myself.

Later, I was grateful for those seminal years of skating, for the ease I still have on the ice, for the discipline I learned working on my jumps and spins, for understanding what it's like to feel scared and skate out on the ice anyway, and for learning to leave the sport at the end of eighth grade when I was done.

I'M NOT AN ATHLETE

By junior high, my timid kid-self turned opinionated. I didn't want to skate anymore. It wasn't cool. Cool kids played soccer or softball. I silently resented my mom for choosing sports for us—we also took ballet—with zero social cachet. I wished she had put me in grittier ones with practical skills, ones that would be social capital in high school.

It felt too late to learn soccer or other team sports, but as I looked ahead to high school, I thought I might be able to catch up with tennis. Our girls' varsity team had recently won the state competition for large high schools. I had watched the players, admiring their strength on the court, their physicality as they ran after shots and fired hard returns. I wanted to be part of it all. I hoped playing on a high-level team would help me get into college.

My friend Sue had started playing, so I asked my mom to sign me up for tennis lessons at our local raquet club, with the goal of making the freshman tennis team. Sue and I entered tournaments in the summer to get ready to play competitively, and I managed to win a game. I left with a T-shirt and a twinge of pride from the proof that I was better than one other player.

The day of the freshman team tryouts, I clung to Sue's side. I didn't know how I would stack up. We lined up against the fence, watching as, one by one, girls went to the baseline and hit ground strokes with the coach.

"Next!" I felt sick, my stomach bottoming out, just like at an ice skating competition.

On the court, I told myself to move my feet, to watch the ball—all of my tennis coach's instructions. I felt crushed when I hit the ball into the net or out of bounds. I worried my serves wouldn't go in.

When I got word I'd made it onto the team, relief swept over me. Sue made it, too. When they handed out uniforms, I couldn't wait to wear the white pleated skirt that signified I was a real tennis player. I had done it; I had made it onto a high school sports team.

I grew into a solid player, in part because I was dedicated, practicing outside on humid, hot weekends during the off-season. I could hit hard when pressed. By my junior year, I made it onto the vaunted varsity team.

I also fell in love with the sport. I felt strong on the green-and-blue courts with white lines, hitting deep forehands into the precise corner I intended or returning a serve with a fiery backhand, sending opponents scrambling around the court. I felt part of something,

hanging out on the bus with my friends and cheering on my teammates during long tournament weekends. I felt cool, wearing the bulky red team sweatpants, then heading out to the court to warm up.

I didn't dare call myself an athlete, however. In my mind, the real athletes ran up and down the basketball court, scored on the field hockey team, or blasted down the track in sprint relays. They owned the hallways with their long, lanky strides. I was a not-so-sporty, school-focused Chinese-American girl, who also played tennis.

"I'm not an athlete," I whispered to myself, even when our tennis team won third place in the state competition.

I didn't know it would be one of the most active periods of my life. Once I moved on to college, the strength I had built over years of

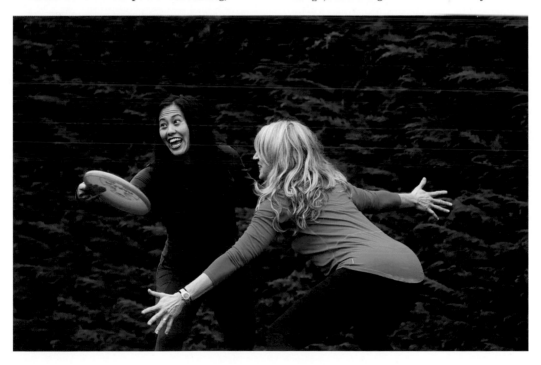

tennis retreated. I walked a lot; dabbled in tap dance, rock climbing, kayaking, and yoga; and pushed myself into feats like a 50-mile hike. But stress and all-nighters ate away at my strength.

As an adult, any lingering athleticism disappeared into the keyboard at work, where I looked at a screen and wrote story after story at the former *Anchorage Daily News*. It vanished into the couch as I sighed and watched television after a long day of writing on deadline. It faded into the elliptical at the gym, where my half-hearted 20-minute sessions were dedicated to preventing additional post-college weight gain.

I will give myself credit for the desire to move. I loved hiking, and I chose jobs near the mountains. I lived in Anchorage for a few years, hiking several times a week in the summer and skate skiing two to three times a week during cold, dark winters to keep my energy and spirits up. I pushed my body because I loved the rush of accomplishment at the summit of a mountain, the connection to mental peace brought on by a 360-degree view, a full day of effort rewarded with pizza and a beer.

I asked a boyfriend once if he thought I was an athlete.

"Not really," he said, shrugging. "Athletic, maybe, but not an athlete."

The comment stung, but he was saying something I already felt inside.

At that time, I worked out primarily to control my weight. I hoped hiking regularly or skiing would drop the fluffy extra pounds that had accumulated after college. Weight loss was the only goal that kept me going to the gym during the spring and fall, transition seasons when I waited until it was time for my favorite outdoor activities again.

LEARNING FROM YOGA

Weight loss was also my underlying driver to do yoga. When I moved to Seattle to work for *The Seattle Times*, I needed a consistent way to move that didn't include the humdrum gym or the traffic battle to hike.

The first time I took a power yoga class, I found my answer.

Back then, the idea of being strong the way I'd felt in high school seemed distant and impossible to rebuild. At 27, I didn't think I could ever reach the strength I once felt on the tennis court, not when my arms wobbled holding a side plank. I struggled when my legs burned in a warrior. I despised the wheel, a deep backbend.

But with steady practice, I lost a few pounds, which motivated me. I went three times a week and was sore every day in between. I limped around, feeling my quads, hamstrings, and glutes screaming at me from new body awareness and being pushed after years of weakness. I wanted to get stronger; I just hadn't realized the road to strength had to be walked with trembling legs.

I also started to absorb what my yoga teachers said about judging my body and myself. I realized I had hated my soft, rounded belly my entire life. In class, I bemoaned my lack of flexibility in a forward fold. I envied my teachers' toned arms and wondered if my arms would ever look like theirs.

For the first time, I saw how hard I was on myself, every day.

In time, my legs quivered less. I could stay upright during balancing poses. I felt comfortable doing handstand hops, even if I couldn't hold a handstand in the middle of the room. I loved workshops where I learned new poses.

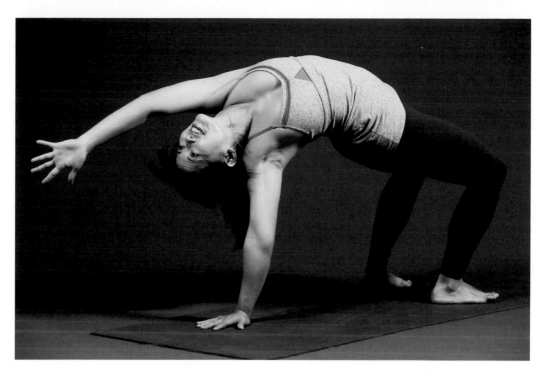

I also was shifting out of the harsh conversations I regularly had with myself. I would start class stressed about my latest story at the newspaper—what I had written or what I'd potentially messed up. I would leave class feeling peaceful, less critical about what had happened that day at work.

Other lessons settled in as I pushed myself into one more wheel or a new pose. Every time I did a pose I didn't want to, just like the first time I'd skated onto the ice to compete as an eight-year-old, my brain was being rewired. Even if a pose looked intimidating or I was tired, I learned to try it anyway.

My new perspective was simple—I can do more than I think I can.

If you asked my friends, people would say I already lived this way. I moved to China to teach English right after I graduated from college. I lived in Alaska for almost four years, braving frigid, dark winters. I covered Congress at 26 years old. At 27 I got a job at *The Seattle Times*, my biggest goal yet.

Then, I left a job in the only industry I had ever known—journalism—to teach yoga. Before I gave notice, I sometimes felt immobilized by worry about leaving behind a steady paycheck, health care, and security, not to mention an underlying concern that I wasn't a very good yoga teacher. Finding the inner strength to walk into my editor's office and tell her I was leaving and then enter a new field where I was reliant on a brand-new skill set radically changed my self-image. I felt I had finally crushed the voice in my head that told me I couldn't do big, challenging things.

FIT FOR LIFE

When the editor of *Pacific NW Magazine*, the weekly Sunday magazine at *The Seattle Times*, emailed me to see if I wanted to chat about a potential writing project, the role of a fitness columnist did not occur to me. Why would it? I had left the newspaper a year earlier to teach yoga. I assumed she wanted to talk about a freelance story.

During our call, she said, "Nicole, we're looking for a fitness columnist. Are you interested?"

I was flattered—and baffled. It seemed ludicrous for me to write about fitness.

"I'm a yoga teacher," I told her. "I don't know anything about fitness."

A yoga teacher is a perfectly good credential for writing a fitness column, she responded.

Was it? I knew how to do warrior poses. I knew nothing about taking a barre class or lifting weights. I didn't even belong to a gym.

The idea, the editor said, was to try new approaches to fitness, take classes, and see what evolved.

I researched fitness columns in other newspapers and couldn't find a columnist who tried a new activity every week; I wondered if there was a reason. I was unsure I could come up with enough ideas to last a year.

But I missed writing. Though I was still enthralled by my new teaching career, my inner writer clamored for me to say yes.

I wrote a column proposal, with ideas including paddleboard yoga, barre classes, and hula hooping. The editors named the column Fit for Life.

The column merged my peculiar mix of skills—writing, a baseline of strength and body awareness, and a willingness to do new things. What I didn't know then was I had signed myself up for six years of weekly reminders that I could do more than I thought I could. I didn't know the column would shatter every internal conversation I'd ever had with myself about my body and strength. I didn't know Fit for Life would redefine my sense of self and reshape my future into one of a forever mover.

All I thought was: Here goes nothing.

CREATING A MOVEMENT-RICH LIFE

Taking weekly classes taught me that if weights or strength were involved, I'd like the class. If there was a competition, I'd want to win. If I was required to run, I'd detest every step, then tell myself afterward it had been good for me.

I learned that my yoga strength could carry me only so far, like when my brain overloaded from dance choreography in a hip-hop class, or I was sore for three days after bouncing on a trampoline for 30 minutes. For the first couple of years, I was sore. All the time.

I became a perpetual newcomer. I took new classes every week; I rarely took any twice. It was comical and frustrating, fun and ridiculous. If you haven't been a newbie in years and are nervous about the prospect of trying something you haven't done before, you are not alone.

I learned to be cool with mastering nothing. As soon as I caught on to a technique in an intro series, the class was over, and I was off to the next. I was forced to let go of concerns about looking foolish, because it was inevitable. You aren't good at something the first time you do it, ever.

The column became the real-life version of a constant internal practice: Do a new thing. Get over yourself. Repeat.

Four years into the column, after I had tried hundreds of classes and learned a tremendous amount about how to recover from intense movement and injury, I was—truthfully—a bit smug. I didn't think there was a whole lot more to discover about movement that I didn't already know. I had done every permutation of high-intensity interval training (HIIT) imaginable. I'd rowed on open water. I'd learned to break-dance, and I'd swung from a trapeze. I'd smiled during swing dance, and I'd swayed my hips to the hula. I'd gotten up at 5:00 a.m. to go to an early morning yoga class followed by a dance party at 7:00 a.m. I'd returned home at midnight after snowshoeing by moonlight.

If you met me at a party and asked if I had tried a particular activity, chances were about 90 percent I had taken a class in it.

ENTER THE SCIENTIST

When I met biomechanist Katy Bowman, who was introduced to me as an innovator in the world of movement, I presumed she would tell me a more detailed version of what I already knew. By then I was subscribing to the approach that had taken root in functional fitness, that the reason to be strong was to carry your kids and live your life. I wanted to be strong! So I, along with so many others at fitness studios, swung kettlebells, did pull-ups, sprinted, and released sore muscles with foam rollers.

I was on the cusp of learning how much I didn't know. I was about to have a massive turnaround in how I approached movement in my life.

An author, teacher, and podcaster, Bowman studies how gravity, pressure, and friction affect people's bodies. What's more, she shows people all the ways they aren't moving, me included. Say what?

After reading her book *Move Your DNA*, I saw all the minutes of the day I didn't move. I had my fair share of hours in a chair hunched over my computer. I added up the minutes spent sitting in my car and the time spent on the couch in the evening as I decompressed or sat at a table eating lunch or dinner.

The more I dug into Bowman's work, which spans multiple books, years of blogging, and a podcast, the more I saw how rarely I walked. My shoes had heels and inflexible soles, keeping my feet from stretching and getting stronger. I hunted for close parking instead of walking a few extra blocks. If I was early to an appointment, I looked at my phone instead of taking a quick walk.

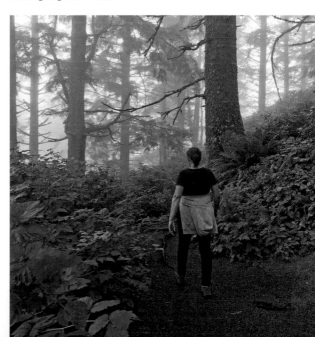

In other words, I was like everyone else I know—sedentary.

Wait a minute. Sedentary?

Because of my one to two hours of workouts a day, I was "actively sedentary," according to Bowman.

Gee, thanks?

But Bowman does not tell people to exercise more. Instead, she prescribes broadening your mind to understand movement and how lack of it affects your hips, back, and shoulders. When you understand how much your body is impacted on a daily basis by choices not to move—enforced all day and everywhere by our sedentary culture—then you can find new ways to add movement back in.

Bowman advocates more time outside breathing fresh air and exposing your body to variation in temperature. Go barefoot on grass and rocks. Sit on the floor instead of the couch or chair. Walk a minimum 10,000 steps per day.

History teaches us healthy movement. In hunter-gatherer times, people sprinted to hunt animals; used their hands, shoulders, and feet to climb trees; and squatted to gather berries from low bushes. Their knees, hips, and shoulders had good range of motion; their feet were supple and strong.

In our modern world, water is piped to our house and food is prepackaged at the store. We sit on a couch, and many of us work at a desk. Sitting on a chair means we skip using ankles, knees, and hips to lower down and get back up. Shoes trap our toes, and elevated heels force us into a position that affects our hips and lower back. We walk less and scramble to find time to exercise.

We have knee injuries, shoulder injuries, and lower back pain. According to the US Department of Health and Human Services, nearly 70 percent of the US population is considered overweight or obese. Bowman says, research has identified sitting and lack of movement as the foundation for almost every physical challenge modern humans face—hip issues, cancer, myopia.

Still, we don't move, not in the ways that will help.

"It's not exercise you need more," she says. "You need to move while getting the rest of your life done."

Many of her suggestions are small and simple, though they were radical to me at first. Slip your shoes off at your desk and stretch your toes. Stand while working instead of sitting. Sit on the floor once or twice a day. Take five-minute walking breaks. Park farther away and walk to your destination.

The US Department of Health and Human Services recommends a minimum 150 minutes of moderate-intensity exercise or 75 minutes of vigorous exercise each week to help avoid diabetes, arthritis, and heart disease. Regular exercisers get an average of 300 minutes per week. But a hunter-gatherer moved 3,000 minutes a week, Bowman writes in *Move Your DNA*.

Bowman wants 10,000 steps to be the baseline, not the goal. She likens exercise to eating something healthy so you can have dessert, but a kale salad doesn't negate multiple crème brûlées. "We can do better than exercise. We need to do *more* than exercise," she writes.

For the first time, my usual one to two hours a day doing yoga or Olympic weightlifting or that week's class for the column felt like underachieving. I took a closer look at the ways I could move more frequently.

I didn't get rid of the couch, but I did build other approaches into my life. I started

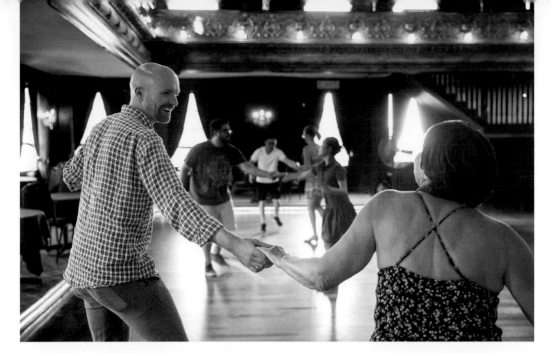

sitting on the floor to work. I rolled out stiff feet and tight glutes while watching television. Fitting in 10,000 steps a day became a daily minimum. To rest my eyes, I looked into the distance whenever I was outside. I've done 20-mile walks with Bowman, who, in addition to being as smart as a whip, is a lively and warm human.

This approach also helps me from getting stuck in the idea I have to "exercise" every day. It's helped me see that when I am sluggish or mentally stuck, all I need is a short walk to invigorate me. If I don't have time for a class, I have other ways to move that are quick and that I can do nearby or at home. Movement has always been a way I connect back to myself, and doing it more throughout the day keeps me steady and anchored.

But my happiest days, my favorite days, still include a fitness class. I go to Olympic weightlifting sessions, I take a dance class, or I do yoga because they make me feel strong, energized, myself. The deeper shift showed

up in the gaps in between, where my new normal and habits changed to walking, to sitting on the floor, to wearing minimal shoes.

Nowadays, I aim to move my body, all day, every day.

WHAT ELSE CHANGED?

For the next two years, I continued taking classes for my Fit for Life column while also working general movement into my life throughout my day, every day. And then, six years after it started, my weekly column ended. A look back at the final class count astonished me—I had tried roughly 300 classes. As I reflected on what I'd learned, I realized how much I had changed in those six years, and especially the final two.

When the column started, I had never tried high-intensity workouts. I didn't know hauling myself up 150-foot trees using climbing gear was possible. I didn't know how much I loved to dance. My original goal had been simple: come up with enough ideas to last a year.

In my early days, I avoided water sports. Now, I relish jumping into the bone-chilling cold of an alpine lake on a hot August day. I like challenging my body to adapt to the dip in temperature. It's refreshing!

I have not gotten over my dislike of running. I gave up making myself enjoy endurance sports and embraced Olympic weightlifting, channeling my fast-twitch muscles into an aggressive hip snap for the snatch and clean and jerk.

I was 34 when I started writing the column, and I closed it out just after my 41st birthday. I was the strongest I had ever been. Even during a short stretch when I had surgery and was limited to walking for eight weeks, I trusted that if I worked hard enough, my strength would come back. Two months post-surgery, I was back on the weightlifting platform and doing handstands in yoga.

I had become a walker. Even now, walking is a nonnegotiable part of my day. Ten thousand steps, or roughly four to four and a half miles, are mandatory. The best days are when I hit 15,000 to 30,000 steps. I have uneven, forested trails nearby and choose the benefit of the soft trails and green canopy over walking on sidewalks during my twice-daily walks with my dog. If my brain stalls at my computer, the best medicine is to get up and walk.

Influenced by Bowman, I switched full-time to minimal shoes, going for flat and flexible in my everyday shoes, stretching my Achilles and feet. Now that I've transitioned from thick hiking boots to barely-there sneakers (see "Hike in Minimal Shoes" sidebar in Month 3), a knee that had nagged me my entire adult life when hiking down steep inclines doesn't even murmur now. I credit my strong, sturdy feet.

Other parts of my life have shifted too. When I travel, I walk no matter what, even in 100-degree desert heat in July in Phoenix. I wear a hat to shield my face and remember my body can tolerate a wide range of temperatures. I always walk whenever I can on vacations.

I never question my strength. I may feel awkward as all get out taking a dance class, or I might dislike an indoor cycling class, but I never wonder if I can do it.

By taking new classes, pushing my body day after day, playing ultimate, or learning to trail run, I've handled whatever was thrown at me. Was it always pretty? Nope. Was I going to master it in one go? No way. Was I going to feel a little silly? Certainly.

Was I going to have fun? Absolutely.

My delight in pushing my body was real, and it still is.

I started the column as a yoga teacher. I ended it as a mover.

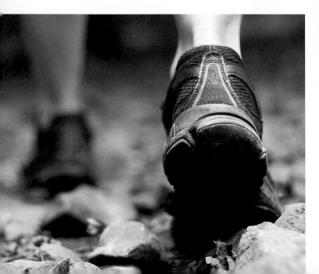

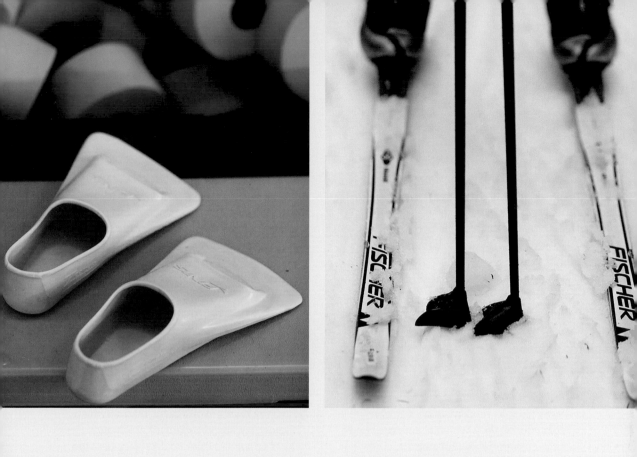

get **moving**

After my last Fit for Life column ran in *The Seattle Times*, I heard from people who'd tried new activities because they followed along as I took on so many myself. I also heard from people who said, "Nicole, I could never do all the things you do."

Oh boy. That statement stirs up the teacher in me. If you want to see me motivated to get other people to move, start by telling me the things you don't think you can do. Tell me the injuries that prevent you from doing an activity you love. Tell me all the ways your schedule and life are too overwhelming to work out.

Tell me, right now. And I'll tell you—it's time to get moving!

Becoming a mover requires you to learn to flex a new type of muscle—the one in your brain. Habits take time to build and discipline to keep in place. I've found the one sure-fire way to make movement part of your life is to do it consistently, which means you need a lot of reminders, plus choosing activities that you *like*. It seems so simple and obvious; it also could change your life.

Inspired by what I learned writing the Fit for Life column and experiencing the life-changing benefits of moving the human body, I designed this book to reset your approach to movement. It will help you shift from thinking that moving your body is a hassle or a burden to seeing it as something that you love, that sparks excitement, that is part of the baseline of your day. Moving is no longer the exception.

If you already love to move, this book is your opportunity to expand your understanding of your own body and movement, and flex the learn-new-things muscle.

What does it take to become a mover? You get to choose. You can move in so many ways.

This book delves into 24 activities that are intended to show you many ways movement is possible while helping you build the habit of movement into your everyday life. You can move on your own, you can move with friends, and you can experience the fun, joy, and challenge of moving with a community. You can see how to add movement to days you don't have time for a class. You decide.

I wrote this book because I don't believe you are physically stuck where you are. I don't believe your injuries are preventing you from moving (that's what modifications are for). I don't believe you will never get stronger. I don't believe you are too busy to move.

I know you can get stronger at any age. Why? I've seen it. I've met a 91-year-old who does aqua aerobics four times a week. I've met the coach for a 79-year-old who became a 12-time world champion power lifter—she started when she was 65 years old. My mother overcame lower back pain in her 70s and walks 10,000 steps a day.

You can get healthy and strong whatever your current physical state. Your body and mind are designed to get stronger and grow. Anyone can learn to try new things, no matter how hard it feels at the beginning.

Not only that, but moving is also the healthiest thing you can do for your brain as you age. In one study, researchers found that a single bout of exercise for participants ages 60 to 80 showed improved cognitive function and memory. Plus, your heart will thank you. A study in the *Journal of the American*

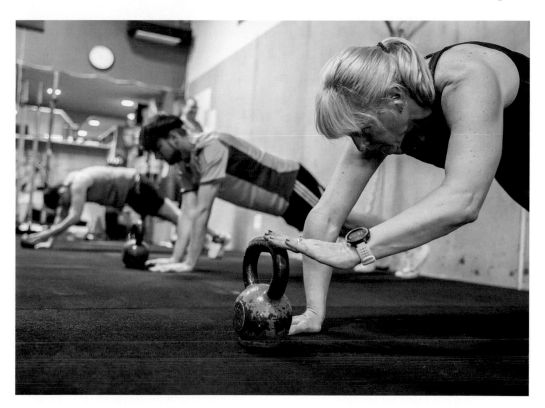

Heart Association revealed that older people who spent less time sitting and more time moving had fewer markers of heart disease. Every 10 minutes spent moving was linked to improvements in heart health, whereas every 10 minutes spent sitting was tied to worse results.

Moving more is essential to living and aging well. Anybody can move more. It doesn't matter where you live, how much you work, whether you can afford to join a gym or take a studio class, or how sedentary your life is right now.

What do you need to become a mover? Your body.

What do you need for this book to work for you? Your body.

What do you need to do to get stronger? Move your body more, and in more ways.

Maybe you moved a lot as a kid and lost your way as an adult. Maybe you never moved much to begin with and are in a deep, committed relationship with your couch. Maybe you've never lifted weights or gone to a dance class. Maybe you have injuries.

You can modify anything. You can always get stronger. You can move more than you are moving right now. The only requirement is a shift in attitude that movement is possible, that you are not stuck where you are, no matter your age or the state of your health.

I wrote this book for *you* to prove yourself wrong. I will be here with you, every step of the way. This book is full of activities and ideas that range in cost and style of movement, with opportunities to journal and reflect on the shift you are experiencing from moving your body more frequently and in new ways. By journaling, you have the opportunity to see how you feel about your body and observe how it changes over time. This book is intended to inspire you to challenge yourself with new activities. There's a reason walking is in the first chapter. Walking is the foundation, the cheapest movement (it's free!), and one that is essential to elevating your health to the next level.

My goal is for you to try every movement at least twice before you move on. That might mean trying each just once a week for two weeks or it might mean adding in a new activity more often than that. It's up to you. After two weeks, switch it up to the second new activity. The key is to pace yourself so you can keep it up for the full year. Each chapter includes a journaling section with charts to help you track and rate your activities.

The only person who can make the change—adding in new activities and pushing you out of what is comfortable—is you. You're the one who has to leave the house, schedule the childcare, find the studio. You're the only one who can do it.

You might be saying to yourself right now that this book is for people who have a lot of time on their hands. Or people who don't have little kids. Or people who already have a good baseline of health or know how to cook and eat healthy meals.

Sure, you can say that. I also know everyone can find five minutes in the day to take a walk or get outside to breathe fresh air. I know everyone can put their phone down and look up at the sky. I know everyone can stretch on the floor while watching television or playing with their kids. If you need accountability, get a couple friends to get on this movement journey with you.

You might say you don't care if you're more active—you just want to lose weight. This book is not about weight loss. Back in the day, when I mistakenly thought weighing 130 pounds would make me happier, I might have said otherwise.

But my happiness has never come from hitting a weight goal. Sometimes, I've lost weight, but that happiness always proved to be fleeting. Over time, I've found that my happiness is rooted in moving my body and finding joy in how much it can do, no matter how I look or what I weigh. The activities in this book are about you putting you and your health first. This book is about setting excuses aside, challenging yourself, and then proving to yourself that you can get healthier and grow.

The world is better when you feel strong. The world is better when you can love and cherish your body. The world is better when you trust your body and ultimately trust yourself. Why? Because when all of those things happen, you are a better human, more balanced and grounded. And everyone around you benefits.

When I started to prioritize movement, my own life shifted. I am a better partner, a more loving sister, a happier daughter, and a better friend when I move. I am smarter and savvier about my work. My relationships and work suffer if I don't prioritize movement above everything else in my day. My mental health suffers. I get grumpy, and I stall out. And so, I move.

Are you ready to move with me?

MOVEMENT ASSESSMENT

How much movement does your body need? It needs to move every day, unless you are a competitive athlete with specific requirements around building strength and rest days. My assumption, dear reader, is that, like me, you are not a professional or competitive athlete. The average person needs to move daily.

Do you move regularly? Or do you think you do?

Start your journey through *24 Ways to Move More* by answering the following questions to get an overall idea of how often you're moving and what that movement looks like. Be honest. These questions will give you a baseline that you can check on again at the end of the 12 months, with additional journaling questions to complete during the year. It will be interesting to see what shifts both physically and mentally through the year. If you're committed to moving more, you need to be aware of where you're starting from and track how far you've come.

How often do you move on a weekly basis?

What types of movement do you usually do and for how long?

What do you like about the types of movement you do right now? Are they fun? Do they give you energy?

If you dislike it, what do you find challenging about the movement you do? Is it the amount of time it takes, the challenge of fitting it into your day, or is it the actual movement that is not motivating?

What were your favorite types of movement as a kid? Do you remember how you physically felt when you did those activities? How did you feel mentally when it was happening? How did you feel when it was over?

Look at the 12 months of movement for this book in the table of contents. Is there at least one movement in there that you did as a kid that you could bring back in?

When you look at the 12 months of movement, are you excited? Or do you immediately come up with a list of reasons why you can't do some of the activities listed there? What are some of the reasons you think you can't do the activities listed?

What attitude shift or intention could you bring to this coming year of movement and trying things you've never done before? What can you be grateful for right now about your body?

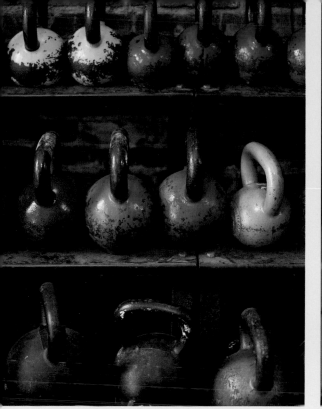
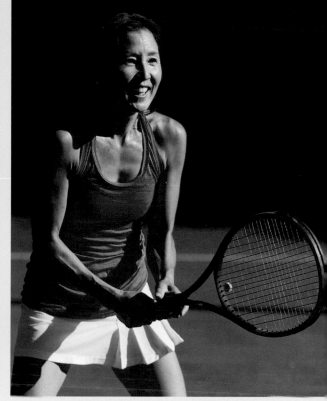

12 months
of **movement**

Before you dive into new movement activities for the next 12 months, be sure you have the information and support you need to take on activities safely.

HEALTHY MOVEMENT

The only person who knows what is going on with your body is you. That said, it takes time to educate yourself about healthy movement, how to differentiate between pain and intensity, and what level of challenge you can handle. Make sure your doctor or a physical therapist has approved you for a new activity before you begin, especially if you are recovering from an injury.

If you are coping with a repetitive, ongoing injury, I can't stress enough how important it is to see professionals. Physical therapists, massage therapists, chiropractors, and acupuncturists are a financial investment, and I can't think of anything more worth your resources than your physical health and recovery. If you have a recurring injury or are physically limited in a way that is preventing you from moving but haven't seen a professional, do that first. See the Recovery sections of this book for more insight into why it matters to see professionals for treating injuries.

NUTRITION AND HYDRATION

What you eat makes a difference in how you feel. When I cut out sugar, processed foods, dairy, and alcohol, I feel better. I don't crash in the afternoon. I feel stronger when I lift.

There are many incredible resources available to help you learn more about fueling your body, particularly when you are moving a lot or doing intense workouts. I recommend getting blood work done by a nutritionist to assess where you are—many folks are lacking in essentials such as vitamin D or iron, which can make a huge impact on how you feel—and, with your nutritionist's support, taking on a challenge like the Whole30 Program or an anti-inflammatory diet to take yourself off processed foods and see how your body feels.

I have tried many diets and cleanses—anti-inflammatory, paleo, Whole30, low carb/ketogenic, the Bone Broth Diet, no dairy, no sugar, no alcohol, doing a cleanse with one day off per week, and so on. It has taken time, experiementation, and working with a nutritionist to find what works best for my body.

My approach is to eat as many vegetables as I can; choose well-sourced proteins and healthy fats; and eat fewer processed carbs, sugar, dairy, and alcohol. I am a stickler about recovery, and I refuel with carbs after I work out. If your heart rate has been elevated for 30 minutes or more, eat some carbs and protein within 30 to 45 minutes to refuel depleted glycogen. Miss the window, and your body turns that fuel into fat, according to my nutritionist. My standby is a banana with peanut or almond butter, but a smoothie with fresh fruit and protein powder or sweet potatoes with some chicken or jerky also work well.

Your nutrition plan will not look like mine, for good reason. You may care to cut out meat. You may want to eat more dairy, or less. Maybe you need to crack the sugar addiction. Perhaps you need to increase certain types of carbs or eat more legumes. Every body is unique.

Do I follow my ideal nutrition plan all the time? Not even close. I love a delicious chocolate chip cookie! But if I feel negative impacts from how I've been eating, particularly if I'm eating out a lot or traveling, I know how to move back to an eating plan that feels good for me. The main point is that what you eat impacts how you feel, in a big way. When you ramp up the amount of movement in your life, it makes sense to take a closer look at your diet.

Lastly, hydration is an essential part of fueling your body. Staying hydrated means carrying water with you wherever you go and adding electrolytes after an intense workout. The average adult body is 50 to 60 percent water. Water helps regulate body temperature, cushion joints, protect your spine, aid digestion, and eliminate waste. If you get dehydrated, your blood volume drops and your heart has to work harder.

FOLLOW THESE BASIC RECOMMENDATIONS:

- Drink 12 to 16 ounces of water as soon as you wake up to make up for water lost overnight.
- Drink an 8- to 12-ounce glass of water at every meal, during exercise, and before you go to bed.
- If you are very active for more than 45 minutes, have a sports drink with electrolytes.
- Get a reusable water bottle and carry it with you so you can drink water throughout the day. Try replenishing by drinking half your body weight in ounces per day, as a baseline (so if you weigh 130 pounds, drink 65 ounces of water per day). Add more with electrolytes when you are active and sweating profusely.

WHY 12 MONTHS AND 24 WAYS TO MOVE?

The first goal of this book is to get you to move more for a full year. Why a year? Because it takes time to make something a habit. The second goal is to encourage you to explore *new* ways to move throughout that year. By taking on something new on a regular basis, you can teach yourself what it's like to try something unfamiliar and challenging with consistency—the pathway to real change.

After taking on a new activity weekly for years, I thought trying two new activities a month felt within reach—so the book offers 24 ways for you to move more over 12 months. Master your new movement practice by doing one activity per week, and repeat every activity at least one more time. While you may fall in love with something right away, remember the point is to keep trying new things. Or you may discover you *don't* love it! That's normal, too. Still, give it a chance. Do it more than once. Muscle memory is magic. The more you practice something, the easier it becomes. You may find that you end up liking an activity you initially hated because you didn't feel like you were good at it.

Keep in mind, too, that if one month's activities feel difficult or frustrating, the next month's are completely new. Be patient and kind to yourself. If you struggle to swim or don't like the dance class, don't give up. Give it a go for two sessions and then move on.

You can start this book at any time, no matter what season you're in. Choose a starting point that works based on the weather, whether it's the middle of winter or the height of summer. Every month is designed to have one activity that can be done outdoors and one that is generally done indoors. The winter sports are grouped together, so if there is snow on the ground where you are, begin there. If you're not up to facing the elements just yet, take on the indoor activity for the month. And some activities can be done no matter what time of year—you can go for a walk in the rain or in the snow! (You always can walk indoors, in a mall for instance, if the weather truly prohibits it.)

This book is designed to be flexible and to accommodate your life. Take a look at your calendar for the month, and figure out when you can schedule trying the new activities. Some take an hour or less, while others are a full-day affair. Part of the challenge is making time to try new things.

Also, if for whatever reason the main activities don't appeal to you, I've included sidebars throughout the book with alternative options. Can't find a hip-hop dance class? Go to tap! Are you struggling with swimming? Check out aqua aerobics. Is it too cold for tennis? Go play squash.

HOW TO MAKE THE MOST OF YOUR 12 MONTHS

Each activity chapter begins with a description of my personal experience with that activity to give you a sense of what it's like as well as the benefits it offers as it adds more movement to your life. From there, the Get Started section helps guide you to begin the new activity, with some quick tips plus basic information on equipment, classes, and costs involved.

If you're already active one to three days a week, the Get Started level should be accessible for you for every activity. Want more? Check out the Challenge Yourself section, which offers three goal levels: Level Up, Reach Goal, and Adventure Goal. Take on a level you feel comfortable with, and build from there. If you're not active, start with walking—go for 15 minutes a day to develop strength over time—then tackle a new activity and set new goals when you feel ready.

Finally, after you've tried a new activity a couple of times, answer the questions posed in the Discovery section. These questions guide you through journaling so that you can document what you've learned, how you feel about your experiences with the activity, and keep track of your progress through the year. Writing about your experience as soon as you can after you've taken a new class will make a difference when you look back over the year and see what has changed. Build in the habit of journaling about movement so you can see for yourself the subtle and big shifts along the way.

The Recovery breaks offer insights on ways to support your body when, for instance, a shoulder, your lower back, or a hip hurts, and I include examples of my own experiences. Recovery techniques apply to more than injuries; all bodies need ways to recover, especially when you take on new activities and challenge your body with new movements.

Turn to Keep It Going at Home for some daily exercises and stretches you can do at home if you don't have time for a class—or even if you do.

The Next 12 Months challenges you to take what you learned over the course of the year and apply it to the rest of your life. You may be surprised by what you learned over those 12 months—and what you want to continue doing or are ready to try out for the first time.

This book closes with a Resources section, which offers additional reading to understand movement more deeply. These include books on mobility and key books by Katy Bowman as well as nutrition resources to enhance what you learn in *24 Ways to Move More*.

LET'S DO THIS!

It will take effort to change your schedule and figure out the logistics needed to start new activities. This is where the internet can come to your rescue. You can find out pretty much everything you need to know about any of the activities in this book online. Almost all fitness studios have robust websites with FAQs detailing what you'll need for class as well as class schedules. If not, go old-school and call for information.

Some activities cost more than others, and each activity chapter lays out what you will need and my best estimate of costs for lessons or classes. Specialized sports need more equipment—winter sports, for example, require more expensive gear and clothing. With most other activities, you can likely make do with what you have.

Don't let equipment dissuade you from doing something you're excited to try. Many times you can rent gear—climbing gyms rent shoes, for example. I recommend renting and

trying an activity before investing in equipment. Be sure you will keep doing the activity, or you may find yourself with a lot of unused new equipment to store!

Class costs vary depending on where you live. In urban centers, a single drop-in class at a fitness studio can run as high as $35. Check around for starter specials, which many studios offer, and don't forget your local community center, which may have exactly the class you are interested in at a much lower cost.

As for choosing which level of class to start, I always recommend an intro or beginner level. When I was writing my column, I almost always started with an intro class. On the rare occasion I jumped into something more advanced, I floundered every time. No matter how strong and experienced you are, you will face a steep learning curve when taking on a new movement. Give your brain time to learn and integrate. Go to a class where the point is to break down the basics and learn that particular movement safely. Learning the basics will make for less frustration and faster growth.

Now that you've absorbed all this information, are you ready? Have you already homed in on the activities that excite you the most—or the ones that make you a wee bit nervous? Good. This book is not designed for you to stay comfortable in the kind of activities you already do. The intention is to move you out of what you already know and to challenge your body and mind in more ways than you thought possible. You're in for a year of incredible growth. Let's do this!

Month **1**

Walking

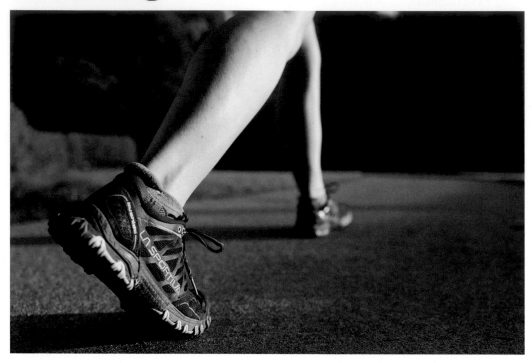

The more I walked, the more I realized how often I had been choosing not to walk. Generally, I drove my car, choosing efficiency—or maybe speed? In the evening, I chilled on my couch, which calls my name at the end of a long day as a place to rest, zone out, and unwind. Plus, it's just sitting there in my living room.

Before I discovered walking as a way to move my body every day, I was proud of how active I thought I was, from yoga to lifting weights to trying new fitness classes. I moved my body for up to two hours daily, far more than most.

Then I read Katy Bowman's book *Move Your DNA* and was promptly toppled from my "I'm so active" high horse. I was exercising, but I wasn't moving the rest of my day, and I definitely wasn't walking much. My step count typically hovered around 3,000 to 6,000 a day, or roughly 2.5 miles, hardly a number to hoot about.

FITNESS DEVICES

I've tried a lot of fitness devices, from trackers to fitness apps. I wanted to know what information they would show me about how much I moved—or didn't move. I also was curious if tracking my physical activity with a fancy gadget would motivate me to move more. My conclusions: Yes to tracking. No to expensive fitness gadgets.

I check my step count daily. My baseline for walking is 10,000 steps a day. I like knowing if I've reached that minimum every day. I've found my phone provides all the info I want, which is how many steps I walk daily. I use a free app that tells me how many times I hit 10,000 steps in a week, month, or year. My phone also keeps information on flights of stairs, but I don't pay much attention to that data. It will track steps even on airplane mode or when I'm carrying it in a bag. The main drawback is I have to have my phone with me, but 90 percent of the time that is already true.

I've also tried gadgets that track not only steps but also a lot of other information while I'm engaged in an activity, and I've briefly been enthralled by a few over the years. Trackers can tell you exact mileage via GPS, show your heart rate, note your current ultraviolet exposure, and calculate how many calories you've burned, and many even come with the added convenience of buzzing when you receive texts. I've worn trackers overnight to assess sleeping patterns. For brief periods, I've worn them for the express purpose of being able to read texts on the device on my wrist instead of picking up my phone.

But, inevitably, all my trackers went by the wayside, some because I grew tired of them and stopped using them, and some due to lack of durability.

Trackers are most useful for runners, who like to know mileage and pace. But for someone like me, who just wants to know how far I've walked in a day, my phone has all the data I could ever want.

Bowman says 10,000 steps is the baseline needed to sustain a healthy body. A study in the *International Journal of Obesity* shows postal workers who walked 15,000 steps a day had no heightened risk for heart disease. Desk workers, however, added risk for heart disease for every hour beyond five that they sat in a day.

Other studies show if you walk briskly for an hour a day, it cuts the effect of obesity-promoting genes in half. It also reduces the risk of developing breast cancer, and it not only reduces arthritis-related pain but it can even prevent arthritis from forming in the first place by strengthening and lubricating joints like your knees and hips. Walking is shown to improve memory and brain function and helps maintain bone density. Walking also helps your immune system. A study of people who walked at least 20 minutes a day five days a week for 12 weeks took 43 percent fewer sick days than those who exercised once a week or less.

The statistics made me want to leap up out of my chair. From Wayne Curtis's book *The Last Great Walk*, I learned that Paleolithic humans likely walked 8 to 12 miles a day, four to six times the distance the average American walks now. Curtis's book follows the journey of the "last great pedestrian," Edward

Payson Weston, who at age 70, walked from New York to San Francisco in 1909. Did you catch that? He was 70 years old. He walked across the entire country!

In between snippets detailing Weston's considerable challenges from weather to footwear to walk 60 miles a day, Curtis digs into the evolution of how humans began to walk, why we walk, and what it does to our bodies and minds. We evolved to walk long distances, and our genetic makeup, locked in thousands of years ago, is based on walking. But in the United States, we are walking less than ever. Not walking "is one of the most radical things we've ever decided to do," Curtis writes.

Not walking also could be unwise. One study found that walking briskly for 30 minutes five times a week reduced the risk of dying prematurely by 20 percent.

Do I have your attention?

The more I learned about walking, the more I felt compelled to walk. Time to get moving.

Squeezing in 10,000 steps, or roughly 4 to 4.5 miles, requires dedicated time to walk. I made it my starting goal. Going out for a walk, even a short one, nets a couple thousand steps, but I also love yoga and lifting weights. I had to figure out how to walk more without taking away time from those.

I needed to get smart about adding in steps.

I looked first at my commute. Hopping on transit was the simplest approach. The 10- to 15-minute walk to my local light-rail station after parking, plus the 10-minute walk from my downtown stop to the yoga studio where I teach and the return walks, would net me 4,000 to 5,000 steps.

I argued with myself to get this new system in place. I was accustomed to curling up over my computer screen right up until the moment I had to hop in my car. I had to build in more time on the front end, since my new plan added about 30 minutes to my commute. It appeared at first that this was going to eat up valuable work time.

The reality was quite different. I saw that I could shift my mindset about taking the train and turn it into productive work time. During my 25-minute ride, I completed writing projects and answered emails; I realized I lost time sitting in my car in traffic. By using transit, I also arrived at my destination with more energy from walking and no stress from traffic. Taking the train also fed into an environmental goal to drive fewer miles.

Soon, I loved my new pattern.

From there, I added in more walks. One day, I walked three miles to an appointment. When I ran out of time for the return, I took the bus. That day, I hit 15,000 steps. On another day, I walked one mile from the light-rail to my gym, did Olympic weightlifting for two hours, and walked another mile afterward back to the station. In the rain. It proved to me I could walk on days I lift or do yoga—and while getting soaked.

I walked while making work calls. If I was 10 minutes early to an appointment, I walked around the block instead of sitting in my car on my phone. I proposed walks with friends rather than meeting for a drink or a meal.

Sometimes, I imitated my mom, a committed walker, and walked laps around my house in the evening to get my last couple thousand steps in. Circling the house felt silly, but I was happy every time I hit that magic five-digit number.

The best days are when I head to the mountains to hike. I reach 15,000 to 30,000 steps on days spent reveling in fresh air, forest trails, and all those glorious steps.

At first, walking 10,000 steps on days I lifted or did yoga exhausted me. Over time, my walking endurance grew. After building it into my routine, I walked my four-plus miles, did other activities, and felt energetic and steady throughout the day. After several months of hitting my 10,000-step walking goal at least five times a week, I was ready for my biggest walking challenge yet.

Katy Bowman had mentioned 20-mile walks to me. She takes these long walks at least once a month and adds them into movement retreats that she leads. The long walk is a lost art in the United States, Bowman says. Americans once took long walks as a matter of course and used to admire great pedestrians. Remember Edward Payson Weston?

I liked the idea, and I was nervous. I wondered if I would make it to the end, or if it would be painful. Still, once the idea was planted, I was not turning back.

On the day of our 20-miler, I met Bowman bright and early on the Olympic Peninsula in Washington, close to where she lives. Bowman mapped out our route and estimated it would take us eight hours with a break. A light mist came down as we collected two other walkers she'd recruited, and we set off.

I asked if I should have trained for the distance. The best way to prepare for a long walk is to do one, Bowman said. Your body uses different muscles at 20 miles than it does at 5 or 10. The long walk is the training. As muscles tire out, your body adapts by relying on different muscle groups. If your feet or ankles are stiff—true for most people—your body

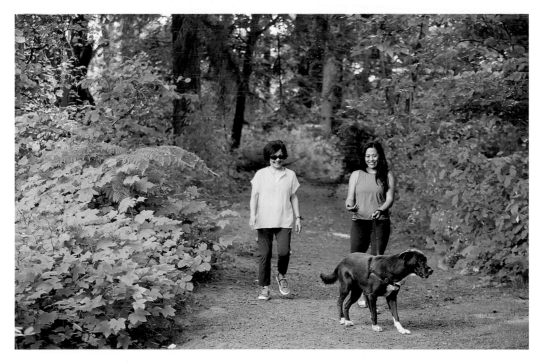

has a hard time getting other muscles to join in, so you might get tired or hurt. The same could happen for knees or hips. It does help to stretch and strengthen your feet and joints over time before your first long walk.

Our fellow walkers were Michael Kaffel, a teacher with Bowman and a veteran of many walks, and his friend Owl. Owl's dog, Ki, walked with us, and Bowman's husband would join us for the last 10 miles.

Worried we might run out of topics to talk about, I'd come up with a list of questions for Bowman, eager to pick her brain. This prep was unnecessary. I didn't even get to my questions because, as I discovered, if you're walking with new people, you'll spend all your time getting to know them.

For the first few miles, clouds spat light rain as we moved along a paved trail close to a highway. Our conversation was nonstop as we shared brief summaries of our life histories, with asides into work catch-up for Kaffel and Bowman. The miles flew as the conversation moved to books. Soon, we were five miles in.

Around eight miles, Bowman moved her backpack to the front of her body. A backpack makes it easier to carry a lot of things,

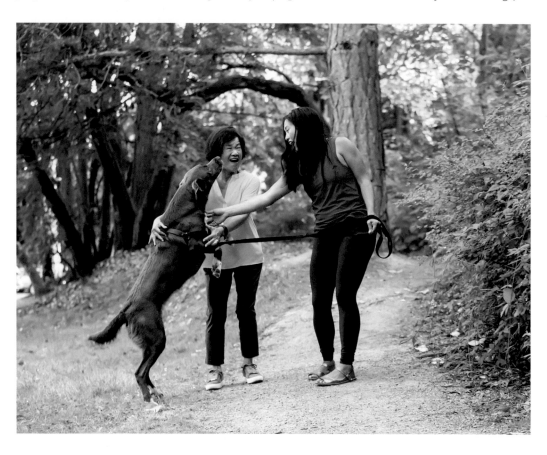

as opposed to carrying things individually in your arms, but your body gets tired holding it. Change position to use new muscles and rest others, Bowman said; it's resting while you move, an idea both novel and sensible. I slung my backpack to one side and noticed the other side relax even as we moved at a quick clip.

To rest our feet from the paved trail, we walked in the grass. Flat ground is easier for fitness, Bowman explained, but more complex terrain is easier on your musculoskeletal system. When you walk on flat ground, you use the same muscles the whole way. On complex terrain, the same concept of alternately resting muscles as you go applies.

We paused to look at a steep ravine filled with lush green forest while we nibbled on cucumber-flavored Indian plum leaf, but our pace otherwise was fast at a little over three miles per hour. At three hours, we had covered 10 miles and arrived at Bowman's house for a mid-walk break.

In her home, Bowman pointed out squishy balls and half-dome rollers in the living room for stretching calf muscles and feet then went to the kitchen to mix batter for crepes. I stretched my legs, squatted, did lunges, and twisted to release tightness in my back. It felt so good to stop walking and stretch.

I thought I would struggle to motivate after lunch, but I felt refreshed and physically good. With Bowman's husband now in tow, we were off to the Olympic Discovery Trail, a 130-mile trail that winds across the Peninsula. Our conversation shifted to Ayurvedic nutrition and acupuncture. Bowman and I chatted about writing books and running our own businesses. We paused when Owl pointed out swarming termites, red ants, or the shape of a vine on a tree. We looked at books in Little Free Libraries. We stocked up on fresh eggs for sale in a cooler by the trail. Bowman took pictures and posted movement tips to her Instagram account.

At mile 16.5, we stopped to stretch. I asked if long walks always pass so quickly. Kaffel, who has done longer ones, smiled and said, "When it's only 20 miles."

Around mile 19.5, my right hip spoke up. It's often tight from an old injury, and it made itself known for the final stretch, aching as I walked. A long walk will show you repetitive movement patterns and weaknesses, Bowman said. Fortunately, we were almost at the end.

As anticipated, our walk lasted eight hours. I thought 20 miles might feel hard, but it didn't. The walk took a long time, but it was nothing compared to the exhaustion I feel from a 12- to 14-mile hike with a lot more elevation. It was just fun—and so simple. For the curious, our walk added up to about 45,000 steps.

I have days I don't reach my daily 10,000-step goal, though it is less frequent since the arrival of my pup, Coco. For her, a 45- to 60-minute morning walk is mandatory, and it's also essential for this dog mom's sanity, so out the door we go. I take Coco on a second walk during the day and continue to leave the car at home or find other ways to get in steps during the day to hit my goal. When I vacation, I make it a point to explore wherever I am by foot to reach 10,000 steps—my biggest exploration triumph was a 25,000-step day.

My goal was to make walking a lifestyle rather than the exception. I can say with authority that walking has stuck around. Want to become a walker? It's as simple as walking out the door.

GET STARTED WALKING

The average person, walking at a smooth rate, typically can cover one mile for every 20 minutes of walking, but slowing down or speeding up works, too. When you're getting started, don't worry too much about number of steps, mileage, or speed. Just go!

Start by taking a 15-minute walk once a day. Make it simple and just head out your front door in the morning before work, take a quick stroll during your lunch hour, or set out in the evening when you get home. Even once around the block is a good beginning.

QUICK TIPS

- Skip new shoes, especially on a long walk. You may end up with blisters, a side effect when skin needs to toughen up. Wear well-tested shoes for your first time out on a longer walk.
- Walking 30 minutes nets you roughly 3,000 steps—and a healthy glow.
- If you're early for an appointment, walk around the block rather than sitting and waiting in your car or an office.

BEFORE YOU GO

Equipment: Comfortable shoes with minimal to no heel that you can wear for one mile or more; breathable clothing, layered, depending on weather conditions.
Cost: Free.

CHALLENGE YOURSELF

Once you master a 15-minute walk each day, consider these additional goals:

Level Up: Twice a week, increase your daily walks to 30 to 45 minutes. Map out all the locations you go to regularly that are within a one-mile radius of your home—the coffee shop, the library, the grocery store—and walk for one of those errands. Add mileage by taking transit to work if possible or by parking farther away from your destination. Add in walking meetings with coworkers.

Reach Goal: Walk 30 to 45 minutes daily. In addition, consider taking another, longer walk once a week, going for 90 minutes or up to three hours. Many city and state parks feature paved paths or dirt trail systems where you can vary the terrain under your feet.

Adventure Goal: Take a 10-, 15-, or 20-mile walk. Use an online map planner to figure out a route. You can do an urban walk, plan a route on a path or trail farther afield, or consider a wilderness hike. Bring plenty of water and snacks, and go with other people to make the walk come alive. Map out bathroom options as well as places to take breaks. Leave details of your plan with a friend or family member for safety.

DISCOVERY: *Walking*

	1ST	2ND	3RD
DATE			
DURATION			
RATING (1 TO 5 STARS)	★ ★ ★ ★ ★	★ ★ ★ ★ ★	★ ★ ★ ★ ★

What preconceptions did you have about walking as exercise when you started taking daily walks? Did you think it would be too easy or you wouldn't have enough time? How do you feel about it now?

How did your body feel at the start of your walking journey? What did you come to enjoy about the physical act of walking and moving your body by taking steps?

When walking, I appreciated less screen time; I made my dog walks screen-free, keeping my phone in my pocket, and tried to focus more on my surroundings and my pup. What did you learn about or observe when you walked? Did you discover something new about your neighborhood?

Cross-Functional Fitness

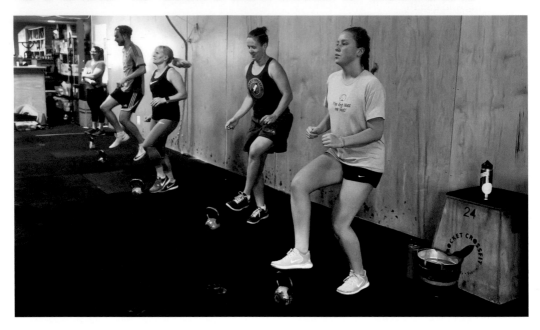

I was suspicious of the enthusiasm. People who do cross-functional fitness, also known as high-intensity workouts or, more popularly as "CrossFit," talk about it in rapturous tones. They blather on about how sore they are, using terminology foreign to us normal folk. They talk about how you can get in the best shape of your life with a 10-minute workout.

Skeptical didn't even begin to cover how I felt. I had no interest in this trend. Nope. Not me. Not in this lifetime.

Then my friend Emily turned. She wasn't just in; she was *all in*. The betrayal!

Emily wanted me to try this high-intensity functional fitness, too. Over dinner, she kept saying how much she loved the workouts and how great the community was. Her gym was close to our respective homes.

I looked into her gym, which utilized the CrossFit brand and required newcomers to take an introductory series that teaches you the exercises and how to safely navigate the rigorous workouts. The price made me gulp—$150 for a month—and this was several years ago. This particular intro series required 12 classes over four weeks—that's three classes

OR TRY . . . KETTLEBELLS

Advocates of kettlebells say you can get stronger than you ever thought possible—including core, leg, shoulder, and grip strength plus general conditioning—by working out with the round-shaped weights with handles that come in various sizes.

I wanted that.

I took a class at a studio that teaches Russian-style kettlebell technique, learning to swing and use the kettlebells for general strength. You train barefoot, which at first seemed dangerous to me, considering that even light kettlebells can hurt if dropped on a bare foot. But feeling your feet makes a difference for technique, according to the trainers, though not all studios train this way.

After a warm-up, we worked a halo, holding a kettlebell in both hands with the handle down and circling the kettlebell around our heads, as close to hair and ears as possible. Halos warm up the shoulder girdle, strengthen the back, and mobilize the shoulders.

We practiced squats, lowering hips toward the floor. Then we learned a hip hinge, folding at the hips, sticking your butt out, and engaging your core. For swings, holding the bell by the handle, we hinged first, dragged the kettlebell back, felt our weight in our heels, then thrust hips forward so the bell floated forward to shoulder height, repeating the swing 10 times, using a breath technique to sniff in and then hiss breath out during the swing.

I struggled with my hip hinge. If you hinge more at the hips, you won't leak power from your core, one trainer said. I lost power at the top of the swing, pushing my hips forward instead of standing up. I muscled my kettlebell up with my shoulders. Clearly, I needed to take this class again.

We also worked deadlifts with heavy kettlebells. I hinged at my hips, squeezed my legs and upper back, sniffed, exhaled, and stood up with my kettlebell.

The goal is to master technique so that you maintain good form even if you swing a kettlebell hundreds of times in one class. I can't wait for the day I master a beautiful kettlebell swing.

a week. That seemed like a lot of money—and time—to commit up front.

Many gyms and trainers offer a variety of multifunctional high-intensity interval training (HIIT) classes. It's often marketed as "CrossFit," a worldwide brand with numerous affiliates, but you can easily find gyms that use similar approaches and get the same results.

This style of training includes bodyweight exercises such as pull-ups and push-ups; weightlifting using barbells (you'll squat and learn Olympic lifting, snatching a barbell from the floor and raising it over your head); cardio, including running, indoor rowing, and jumping rope; and gymnastics-style movements, such as muscle-ups (swinging up onto a set of hanging rings) and handstands.

In a HIIT workout, the movements typically change every day. Some days are technical, when you focus on a snatch for 30 minutes before doing an intense 10-minute workout. Other days, you'll do a "chipper," moving for 40 minutes between a power clean (an Olympic lift), running, kettlebells, and throwing a medicine ball overhead at a wall, for example. The high-intensity part of the workout comes from the nonstop element; you do the pre-scribed movements until time is up or you've completed a set number of reps.

The goal is to improve overall fitness and home in on areas you can get stronger. You'll find movements you love and ones you struggle with. If you've never done strength training, you may be surprised at how quickly you progress. If you want to improve your cardio and aerobic capacity, have no fear—your body's ability to get oxygen to your muscles will skyrocket.

Once you get more experienced in cross-functional fitness, the benefits increase, stud-ies have shown, with better aerobic capacity and more strength. Although you may hear about potential injuries, research has shown that the frequency of HIIT-related injuries is consistent with those associated with any type of fitness activity.

I was lured in by HIIT's short workouts. Emily was effusive about how efficient the workouts were, and I loved the idea of pushing hard for 10 minutes—though I would soon find out many workouts lasted longer than that. I also hadn't joined a new fitness community in years, and my interest was piqued when Emily described the program's outgoing, encouraging culture. I wanted to meet new people, both to work out with and to build new friendships. Her CrossFit gym sounded like a jump-start for body and soul.

On the first day of the intro class, our trainer, Jenelle, eased us in. We learned proper squat technique and how to go deep into a squat by dropping our hips below our knees, and we worked on push-ups, modi-fying as needed with knees down. We made pull-ups easier by attaching a stretchy band to a bar and stepping into the bottom to get some needed lift up over the bar. I hadn't

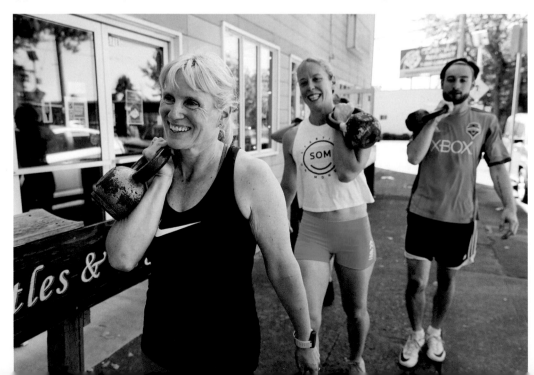

attempted a pull-up in years and relied on the boost from the thick rubber band.

We did a timed workout—a HIIT staple—with a 200-meter sprint, running on pavement outside and around the block, followed by three rounds of air squats (squatting your hips below your knees), push-ups, and ring rows (holding a set of rings, walking your legs forward so your body is diagonal to the ground, and pulling your chest to the rings, a modification to build shoulder strength for pull-ups). We finished with a final sprint. Loud music pounded throughout the workout, and Jenelle shouted encouragement. I was breathing hard, but I liked it. We recorded our times in journals at the end of class.

I walked out of the gym energized by doing the workout and by meeting new people who lived close by and were intrigued by HIIT. I was excited about the next workout. Maybe it was the endorphins or an adrenaline buzz, but I almost skipped to my car.

Who was I? All it took was one workout to become one of *them*?

I thought about the workout for the next two days and couldn't wait to go back, despite the soreness in my shoulders from the push-ups and pull-ups. I was excited every time I got to class; three times a week didn't feel like enough.

As we progressed through the intro series, the workouts increased in length and intensity. The combination of cardio with strength training is brutal, if effective, even when the cardio is a short 200-meter sprint. I hate running, though I discovered I was a decent sprinter. But running tested my lungs; by the third round of sprinting, rowing, or jumping rope combined with pull-ups, squats, or lunges, I was gasping.

Finally, we had a workout with "no cardio." We learned to do wallballs—taking a large, heavy medicine ball, squatting while holding the ball, and then standing up and heaving it up above a marked height on the wall.

Yes! I thought when I watched the demonstration. I was gonna love this.

Perhaps it was best I went in blind. Five rounds of wallballs combined with push-ups and pull-ups later, I was on the floor, panting (collapsing on the dirty gym floor became the norm; you get used to being grimy). In cross-functional fitness, the running joke is: Wanna do cardio? Lift faster.

I had heard from the internet that some gyms throw you in too hard, too fast, and I didn't know if I would like the intensity. The intro series was a soft entry; I never felt overwhelmed, an indicator of a good gym.

HIIT also gave my competitive side a new outlet. It's never far below the surface, but I hadn't taken on a competitive physical activity since high school. With timed workouts, I wanted to come out on top every time. I watched the clock and other athletes, talking myself into moving even when I felt like another burpee was impossible.

After my intro series was over, I wanted to keep going.

I got strong fast doing cross-functional fitness, a common result when you go from no weightlifting to lifting three to four times a week. While I'd once thought I hated weightlifting, I found that what I actually hated was lifting weights on a machine. I fell in love with the dynamic movements of Olympic weightlifting.

I also discovered that it takes time to develop the endurance and capacity for the intense workouts, and I was sore a lot, sometimes hobbling for a couple of days. But I was amazed to see how much stronger I got.

With the ever-changing workouts found in HIIT, it's difficult to avoid exercises you dislike. It took me a year to do more than one double-under in a row, whipping the jump rope around twice on one hop. I despaired when the options were a 5K run or a 5K row on the rowing machine. Throwing myself to the floor and hopping back up to jump and clap overhead for a burpee felt like the death of me.

It helps when others tackle a workout with you. I bonded with many members of my classes over workouts. As I got to know them, I figured out which people I was on par with physically. At night, I was glued to Facebook, where coaches posted workout times from the day, scrolling through everyone's results. As I've said, I'm competitive.

I struggled for a while between pushing myself and overextending my body. My competitiveness got the best of me one summer,

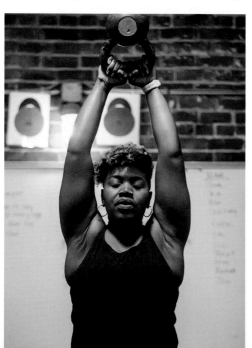

and I tweaked my shoulder. I took the injury seriously and scaled back until my shoulder healed. I modified my workouts, using a thicker band for pull-ups and reducing weight on my lifts. I found that even modified high-intensity interval workouts produce sweat and can cause post-workout collapse.

More importantly, HIIT had a huge impact on my perception of my own strength. Prior to the training, I couldn't do a pull-up, or even come close, whereas I now consider doing one or two pull-ups a baseline.

Cross-functional fitness also shifted my approach to nutrition. I had done simple cleanses before, such as eliminating sugar or alcohol for a month. Otherwise, I assumed I ate well. Then I did my first-ever Whole30 nutrition challenge—hosted by my gym—and cut out sugar, processed carbs, dairy, alcohol, and grains. I realized that a diet packed with good protein and vegetables stabilized my energy and made me feel stronger during workouts.

The workouts became a staple in my life. For the first time ever, I loved going to the gym and pushing my body in new ways. I loved lifting heavy weights. It was a thrill to go to fitness classes and see how much stronger I was and how much more endurance I had.

Most HIIT programs emphasize meeting everyone at the start of class, cheering folks on until they finish, and building community. I loved giving people high fives as they ran past me and grimacing with my friends when workouts felt harder than I ever thought possible. I watched people of all shapes, sizes, ages, and fitness levels come in and get fit and strong.

For a friend's 40th birthday, I went to a workout called the Fatal 40. Tons of us packed the gym, sweating through squats, power cleans, pull-ups, push-ups, burpees, and running. During one set of 40 burpees, I was exhausted. I didn't want to do any burpees, let alone 40; I had a few moments when I was ready to skip the burpees to finish. But then I remembered the only goal was to keep going—always my main mindset in classes. I saw other people gritting it out. I shook it off and did all the burpees.

As always, I made it to the end.

GET STARTED WITH CROSS-FUNCTIONAL FITNESS

There may be multiple HIIT programs, like CrossFit, near you. First talk to folks who work out there to get a sense of whether it's the right fit for you. Look at gym photos and see if they reflect a variety of ages, races, and body types. See if they have a structure for new members to onboard. Go in and see how you are treated. Then take the required intro class or a one-on-one with a trainer to learn the basic movements.

Once you're working out, get to know the people sweating next to you. It makes a huge difference to create a community that holds each other accountable and cheers each other on.

BEFORE YOU GO

Equipment: HIIT-specific shoes, useful for both running and weightlifting. Down the road, you may want to invest in a pair of lifting shoes. Wear sweat-wicking workout clothes.

Cost: Monthly fees depend on the gym, ranging from $90 to $300 per month at city gyms.

QUICK TIPS

- Some gyms post daily workouts online in advance. Don't let a particular workout dissuade you from going to the gym that day. The point is to vary your movements. Challenge yourself with workouts you may not want to do.
- If your gym hosts nutrition challenges, participate in one to learn more about how what you eat has an impact on how you feel.
- Give yourself time to recover between classes. It's a lot of new movements at a higher intensity than you may be used to. You may feel quite sore.

CHALLENGE YOURSELF

Your intro series may cover a full month, depending on your gym. If not, consider adding the following goals:

Level Up: Work on mobility outside of class, such as using a foam roller on hips or glutes, or stretching your feet (see "Recovery: Myofascial Release"). This also is useful for recovery in between intense classes.

Reach Goal: Take a cross-functional fitness class one extra time per week. Work on foundational skills, such as a pull-up or double-unders. If your gym posts the workouts online, see if you can go without looking at the workout of the day beforehand so you don't skip workouts you dislike.

Adventure Goal: Sign up for a cross-functional fitness competition. Do it with others at your gym for the fun and challenge of it.

DISCOVERY: *Cross-Functional Fitness*

	1ST	2ND	3RD
DATE			
DURATION			
RATING (1 TO 5 STARS)	★ ★ ★ ★ ★	★ ★ ★ ★ ★	★ ★ ★ ★ ★

What preconceptions did you have about cross-functional fitness (or HIIT, CrossFit, etc.) before deciding to take a class? Did you think it was cultlike or that there was no way you would do it?

What did you discover about cross-functional fitness after taking a class? What did you learn about yourself by doing the workouts?

What was the most challenging part of a high-intensity interval workout? Why?

What have you discovered about your perception of your own strength and health since trying HIIT? How has your body changed since taking classes?

Month **2**

Swimming

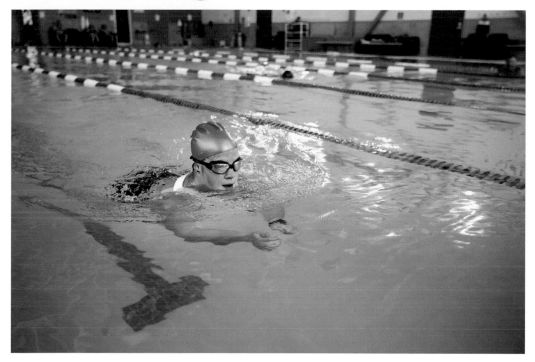

"Feel the viscosity of the water," coach Kyle Johnson encouraged as I stood in the water in the outdoor pool, swiveling side to side and letting my hands float in the vivid blue water. "Notice how the water moves off your body and skin. Let the water slide off your arms and torso."

I felt like I had entered some alternate aquatic universe that had nothing to do with swimming, except that I was standing in a pool wearing a bathing suit.

I'd learned to swim when I was a kid and took regular lessons at our neighborhood outdoor pool. Back then, I practiced breathing to the side during the crawl, loved the slower breaststroke, and enjoyed the languorous sidestroke. I hated the days we went for the backstroke, closing my eyes and trying not to choke when water splashed over my face.

I spent most of the summer biking to the pool, where my friends and I leaped off the diving board, dared each other to go off the high dive, practiced forward and backward somersaults in the water, and made faces at each other underwater. I could play in the pool all day.

But as I got older, the pool no longer called to me as other activities beckoned. Those hot summer days with friends felt like a long-ago memory, and I rarely swam. I can't pinpoint the moment, but it probably started with junior high and feeling awkward about how I looked in a swimsuit. I also dreaded getting into cold water and hated getting my hair wet and having to shower afterward. Yup, it was a long list.

I pushed swimming out to the fringes of my life. I preferred water sports where a paddleboard or a kayak was involved so only a small part of me ever got wet. For many years, I didn't jump into green-blue alpine lakes even after a long, sweaty hike, no matter how refreshing my hiking buddies said it was or when they argued that a cold swim was so good for my lymphatic system. I retreated, stubbornly watching from the shore as people jumped in, shrieking. When they emerged, soaking and joyfully refreshed, I was happy I was still dry.

My dislike of water made me a great candidate for working with Johnson, an accomplished triathlete and outdoor swim coach. His expertise is getting people comfortable with the water and swimming after years out of the pool. Johnson often works with adults who've tried learning to swim from online videos, but it's not an intuitive way to understand how water works, he explained.

Swimming is known for its cardiovascular challenge and full-body workout while at the same time being gentle on your joints, and it requires strength and flexibility to do well. It makes a difference to start out slowly and, as you get stronger, work up to more time in the pool. Even those in the best of shape must adapt to moving in the water, which uses different muscles. If you're coming back to swimming, you'll likely feel exhausted after a short swim, no matter how fit you are.

Johnson watched me swim and zeroed in on why I disliked swimming; I was stiff and uncomfortable. I was forcing my way through the water, wasting energy and fighting it with every stroke instead of moving with it. "Water always wins," he said.

Instead of working on form and technique, Johnson teaches his swimmers to pay attention to the sensation of the water first. Your body is used to gravity on land, so when you change the pull of gravity on your bones and tissue, it can feel weird. In the water, your brain must learn to work with water's buoyancy, with its lightness and instability and rhythm.

Getting comfortable in the water is key to not feeling overwhelmed. Shift your focus away from being afraid or nervous and into the sensory part of your brain and body, and you can adapt faster—and perhaps even start to like the water.

As a yoga person, I understood the concept of shifting my focus from the mental chatter in my mind to the physical sensations in my body.

In theory.

To warm up, I swam in a crawl across the pool while Johnson watched my form. I was soon out of breath and thought crossly that swimming is hard and exhausting. Also, the pool was cold. I was full of my usual swimming complaints.

I had not mastered focus on sensation yet, not while swimming.

Johnson must have noticed I was irritated. Were my facial expressions that obvious?

He slowed it down and brought in simple breathing exercises. I stood in the water, wrapped my hands around my ribcage, and breathed deeply, concentrating on the exhale. We did this several times, with me feeling the widening of my ribs on an inhale and the contracting of muscles and bones on the exhale. I started to calm down and relax into the sensation of the water. I stopped caring—at least for a moment—that I was cold.

For my next lap, I paid attention to my breath. That's it. I didn't have to focus on anything else, including form. All I had to do was breathe deeply into my ribs while swimming a lap. I wasn't supposed to think about whether my arms or legs were moving the right or wrong way.

The breathing exercise helped me relax, and I shifted into the physical feeling of doing a crawl. I could feel tension melt out of my shoulders as I swam.

Next, I floated facedown in the water in the deep end, muscles and joints loose. As I floated, I saw my legs sink down toward the bottom of the pool, common for people tight in the shoulders and hips. My bones must be heavy, I thought; maybe I don't float.

With very few exceptions, you do, Johnson said. "Pay attention to the buoyancy in your legs and notice the relative heaviness of your pelvis and neck. Feel where gravity pushes down on your body in the water,"

OR TRY . . . AQUA AEROBICS

I felt calm before my first aqua aerobics class. I had excessive confidence, having spent countless childhood hours in a swimming pool.

At the pool, an older man named Angelo told me I might want a belt to keep afloat in the deep end. I was slightly offended but grabbed a belt, secured it around my waist, and eased into the water. The belt keeps your head above water, but just up to your chin. I gurgled, trying to tread water and not go under.

Our perky instructor, Lynelle, showed up at the side of the pool. I soon realized I could not keep up with her poolside tempo. My legs flailed under me, and I was thankful no one could see. Add the sensation of sinking, even with my belt, and I soon gasped for breath.

After 20 minutes of straight cardio, our legs and arms churning, we each grabbed a noodle. I was relieved. We held them like bicycle handles and propelled our legs underwater. Then we learned the pièce de résistance—stand on the noodle and balance. I tried to get both feet on the noodle but toppled over.

Still, I loved the buoyancy of my noodle. When Lynelle had us grab dumbbells, I was reluctant to put it aside.

The dumbbells also provided lift. I pushed them underwater for arm resistance, and I bobbed up. I caught my breath and even enjoyed class.

To close, we swam across the pool as fast as possible. Angelo kicked my butt. Aqua aerobics confirmed I've got some work ahead of me to get stronger in the pool.

he coached. "It's different from your body on land."

Next, he had me concentrate on lengthening my neck, stretching through my head as I swam and lifting my head to stretch my neck even more while breathing, and on moving my legs from my stomach, using hamstrings and glutes so that my legs undulated like "tree branches." He told me to try not to kick in a disconnected, jerky, and inefficient fashion—although when coaching, Johnson talks about moving your legs, not kicking.

I tried it all. I tried to feel my core. I tried to imagine my legs undulating like tree branches. I tried not to kick. Then, I sputtered as I tried to do everything at once. I could tell my brain was going into overload from all the new information.

My sputtering signaled it was time to do a breathing exercise called alligator. Johnson had me lower into the water with my mouth open until water filled half of the cavity. You can breathe through your mouth, even with water in there. I was mesmerized. It's possible I learned this in swim classes as a kid and forgot. As an adult, it was a revelation.

The exercise also ensures you don't panic when water gets into your mouth while swimming. As I practiced, my mouth half full of water, I was inwardly freaked out, even though I was breathing just fine.

I got Johnson's point. There's nothing to panic over. Stay calm.

On the next lap, I stopped worrying about water in my mouth. I relaxed my muscles, letting myself feel more buoyant and lighter in the water. I played with undulating my legs and was starting to feel like I was one with the water, rather than fighting it to make sure I didn't go under.

It took only a half dozen exercises before I was ready to move on to form. I started with diggers, swiveling from side to side while standing in waist-deep water and letting my arms flow through the water as I swiveled. I relaxed my arms, allowing them to swoosh and curl through the water in a natural sway similar to how they move when I walk. You want to incorporate that natural feel when you swim, Johnson said.

During the next lap, I focused on my arm curve I felt while swiveling, and Johnson could see clearly that my stroke had changed after the simple arm exercise. I used fewer strokes to get to the other end of the pool. I was more excited that I wasn't gasping for air by the end of the lap than I was about form.

Lastly, I practiced dolphin jumps—standing in the shallow end of the pool, jumping up into the air and down to the bottom, and using my hands to push back up again to get a sense of momentum, speed, and the natural forces of buoyancy and gravity. These were fun and energetic. I loved leaping into the air and diving down and pushing back to the surface. It reminded me of doing somersaults and handstands in the pool as a kid, always my favorite part of being in the water.

With this last exercise, my lesson was done.

Johnson said his main goal is to get swimmers out of their own way. "I remove the clutter and get them back into their body," he said.

After the hour-long session, I could see the liquid light. Swimming can rule.

If you'd like to add swimming to your workout routine, whether you're new to the sport or coming back to it after a long hiatus, you'll find it takes time to get into swimming shape. Taking classes is always the best option if swimming is new to you or even if it's been many years since you've been swimming. Technique likely has evolved since you last swam regularly, and it's a great time to brush up on your skills and learn new ones. As with any sport, consistency is key to making it easier, more enjoyable, and a boon to your overall health and fitness.

Most cities and many other communities have affordable public pools, so if the pool is beckoning, why not heed the call?

GET STARTED SWIMMING

Check out your local pool's schedule of classes, open swim, and lap times, and carve out 20 to 30 minutes for a session where you get in the water, do some breathing exercises, and start to work with a kickboard or swim a few laps. Go twice a week for a couple of weeks to get started.

BEFORE YOU GO

Equipment: Bathing suit, towel, goggles (optional), bathing cap (optional).
Cost: Costs vary from pool to pool. Public pools typically charge adults around $5 for an open swim session. Check your local pool for swim rates, classes, and schedules.

CHALLENGE YOURSELF

Once you've gotten comfortable in the pool and can swim a few laps without stopping, it's time to work on new skills and challenges, like these:

Level Up: Create a training plan for yourself, such as five 100-yard sets with a break in between. You can time yourself for each set, or allow yourself a limited break, such as 30 seconds, between each set.
Reach Goal: Check to see if your pool has master swim classes, which are essentially set swim workouts. These are ideal once you're comfortable with a crawl, backstroke, and breaststroke and can potentially butterfly. You'll swim with other people working on the same series of strokes, distance, and time.
Adventure Goal: Swim in nature. Go to a local beach or lake to swim. Challenge yourself to focus on your breath and stay relaxed in the water.

QUICK TIPS

- Get comfortable in the water first. Do some breathing exercises; then grab a kickboard and warm up. Once you're ready, move into a crawl.
- Mix up your strokes. Do a backstroke and see how it feels to look up at the ceiling or sky while using dividers to keep yourself going straight. Slow down with a breast stroke, which gives you a great view of where you're headed and still challenges your body.
- Don't go too hard, too fast. Cap your time and take breaks between laps.
- During scheduled lap swims, most pools don't allow people to stand or wade. The lanes are marked by speed, but speed varies depending on who shows up on any given day. Slow lanes are at the edges of the pool, and the fastest lanes are usually in the center. Pick the right one for you.

DISCOVERY: *Swimming*

	1ST	2ND	3RD
DATE			
DURATION			
RATING (1 TO 5 STARS)	★ ★ ★ ★ ★	★ ★ ★ ★ ★	★ ★ ★ ★ ★

How did your body feel when you first got into the pool? When was the last time you went swimming, and how did it feel compared to what you remember?

How did you feel physically during your first session in the pool? What changes did you notice after swimming a few more times?

Did you notice any change in your excitement or interest in swimming after going a few times?

If you went for the Adventure Goal, what did you observe about the differences swimming in a pool versus in nature? What did you discover about yourself when you took on a new swimming environment?

Hip-Hop Dance

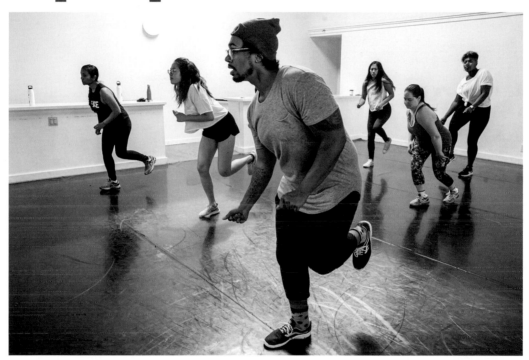

Two days after a hip-hop dance class, I couldn't get Rihanna's song "Numb" out of my head. The song is catchy. I also heard it at least a dozen times in one hour. If only the nifty, complicated dance moves I'd tried to learn along with it had embedded themselves in my body the same way.

I got the idea to take a hip-hop class from an acquaintance who was head over heels for hers and loved how much fun she had dancing. Dance helps with mood and self-confidence, and it reduces stress. Studies show it is central to aging well, from the brain challenge to the balance and focus required, regardless of style. I've met dancers aged 2 to 102, and while you can dance for fitness, for many people, that's secondary to the other benefits—self-expression, joy, community. While dance has clear physical benefits, the mental and emotional ones run deep.

Still, I was nervous about taking a dance class. My brain and body coordinate well most of the time; the main exception is learning dance choreography. I love the challenge, even though I flounder every time my arms, pelvis, and feet must move in different directions at the same time and to a specific beat. But the all-levels hip-hop class at a local dance studio looked like it catered to both dancers and untrained dancer types like me, so I decided to give it a whirl.

Hip hop dance is a street dance that evolved from hip-hop culture, inspired by complex rhythms and movements from African dancing. It features freestyle, or improvisational, dance.

My packed class started off high energy. With some students sporting cool street sneakers and stylish outfits, it felt like a brightly lit club. After a series of stretches and fast-paced core work, Jaret took us through dance progressions, teaching us the sequences first on a slow count, then speeding it up. I had a blast with these simple progressions.

Next step: learning the choreography. Jaret teaches new choreography every two to three weeks, and we were in week two. Jumping in late didn't bode well for my brain and body, which took their sweet time picking up dance moves.

The choreography started simple and slow. We swung our arms in circles. We spun 270 degrees on the balls of our feet. We rolled our hips. We jabbed our pointer fingers in different directions. We grabbed collars. We popped bent elbows side to side. We popped knees for emphasis.

But let's be real—Jaret popped elbows and knees, and so did many folks in the rest of the class. I was trying to pop, but my pops lacked sharpness and were often behind the beat.

Then Jaret took it up to speed. I tried to keep up as Jaret's spiked hair bobbed furiously, and he shouted, "Hit, hit!," "Step ball change!," and "Boom boom!" I was happy he yelled out what the moves were, even as I lagged behind.

Jaret added eight counts of choreography at a time, working us slowly through each full count, bringing us up to tempo, then moving into a new eight count. New dance moves flooded my brain. Sometimes I could remember all the details in an eight count and do them in order. I occasionally anticipated the next set of eight. I gasped, giggling each time he added more moves. It was fine when it was slow, but the faster the tempo went, the harder it got.

And he kept adding more steps. And more. And more.

My brain felt like a circuit board that had gone bust and was now shooting black smoke into the air.

I tried to signal Jaret telepathically—I had reached my dance choreography limit. Time

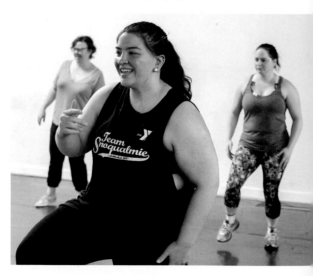

OR TRY . . . TAP DANCE

As soon as I heard the sharp taps of my teacher's shoes on the hard, wood floor, I was smitten. I love how joyful people look when tapping, clickety-clacking their feet with splashy arm moves and huge smiles.

But first, I had to learn technique. I had taken a few tap classes in college, and I remembered footwork was one of my weaknesses.

Teacher Steven seemed confident I would be okay in beginner tap. We tapped out ball-heel to start, and I got in satisfying clacks in my borrowed shoes. After getting a basic rhythm in our feet, he had us reverse.

For shuffles, I brushed the ball of my foot forward and back for a softer shushing sound. My right foot cooperated on this move, but my left foot refused to obey my commands to shuffle, particularly at a fast pace. We also practiced the cramp roll, or ball-ball-heel-heel. It made one of my favorite high-speed tap sounds, with four fast clicks in a row.

For choreography, I crossed my fingers. In isolation, I could do individual steps, but in tap, anticipating the next step is essential. Tap requires balance on the ball or heel of one foot almost the entire time. I tried to balance and also think ahead.

After several practice rounds, I felt comfortable looking away from Steven's feet and added in some jazzy arm moves for flash. When all the dancers dialed into the choreography and tapped in sync, our taps reverberated through the room. I loved it.

When I got home, I found my college tap shoes. It's time to dance.

to shut it down and retain the moves I had successfully programmed into my brain. Put in any more, and the ensuing meltdown was not gonna be pretty.

I was sorry to see that Jaret did not receive my messages; he kept going. He threw in more spins, extra stomps, and a few shoulder snaps. The repetition, at least, helped me slip in one or two correct pops each time.

Finally, he split the class into groups of four. It was our moment to take the floor in front of the class and shine. Or, in my case, survive.

Dancing in front of everyone was easier than I thought it would be, with dancers cheering each other on. I remembered a chunk of steps and had fun sweating, laughing, and popping body parts I didn't know

could pop. It was only a matter of time till I could master fluid hip rolls.

After class, I couldn't stop talking about how much I loved it. I was was even more thrilled when I had time to go again, though I took it down a notch with an intro class. I wanted to catch more moves.

In this class, teacher Michael had us work first on getting comfortable dancing by lining us up to dance freestyle across the room. We moved to the beat, unencumbered by any rules. Then he added in some structure—dance four counts moving your upper body, four counts lower body. Dance as stiffly as you can. Dance sensually. At times, I giggled and felt embarrassed. But I also knew the only way to learn was to do it, so I went all in every time.

Michael gathered us back for choreography. Rolling your body is an essential part of hip-hop, and we worked on a full-body roll, starting with our heads, moving down our spines to our legs. My rolls were jerky rather than fluid like an ocean wave, but I liked trying.

The intro choreography was simple, at first. I loved the Bart Simpson, jabbing my elbows side to side; I was delighted when we did the running man. Michael showed us how to bounce and lean our upper bodies away, a twist that gave the move a quintessential hip-hop vibe.

But as the tempo sped up and he threw in a hop that started on an offbeat, a familiar feeling took over—my brain was maxing out. We did a hop side to side that started on an offbeat, which I hit on the correct beat once in 20 tries.

By the time we broke up into groups, I was laughing, messing up, and just trying to keep up with the choreography.

Our 90 minutes flew by. It confirmed what I'd felt after my first hip-hop class—I'm better at choreography than I give myself credit for; when I dance, I smile nonstop; and I need to practice. I can't wait to go back.

GET STARTED WITH HIP-HOP DANCE

Find an introductory hip-hop dance class and commit to going once a week. Check local community centers for more affordable options or your local gym for classes. If you live in a city, look for dance studios that offer classes. If the class is working through a series of choreography, keep going back. You'll build on what you learn each week and may be surprised by how much you progress.

QUICK TIPS

- Don't get too hung up on getting the exact moves down. Have fun while you dance.
- Ask your teacher if you can record the full dance choreography so you can practice at home.

BEFORE YOU GO

Equipment: Sneakers and comfortable clothes to move in—you'll probably sweat!
Cost: Class fees vary depending on location, ranging from $10 to $25.

CHALLENGE YOURSELF

Once you've gotten comfortable with learning dance choreography, there are many fun ways to ramp up your dance skills. Try these:

Level Up: Go to a hip-hop dance class twice a week and practice your choreography at home.
Reach Goal: Join an intermediate or advanced hip-hop class, taking on more difficult choreography.
Adventure Goal: Sign up for a performance. If you take a hip-hop class at a dance studio, they may hold regular performances showcasing their students. Challenge yourself to get on a stage!

DISCOVERY: *Hip-Hop Dance*

	1ST	2ND	3RD
DATE			
DURATION			
RATING (1 TO 5 STARS)	★ ★ ★ ★ ★	★ ★ ★ ★ ★	★ ★ ★ ★ ★

How did you feel the first time you went to a hip-hop dance class? Were you nervous or excited? Why?

What did you discover about your coordination and ability to try something new in the class?

What did you learn about muscle memory during the first class? What did you discover about it by the end of a month?

What did you learn about how dance makes you feel in your body and mind and how it affects your energy level?

Hiking

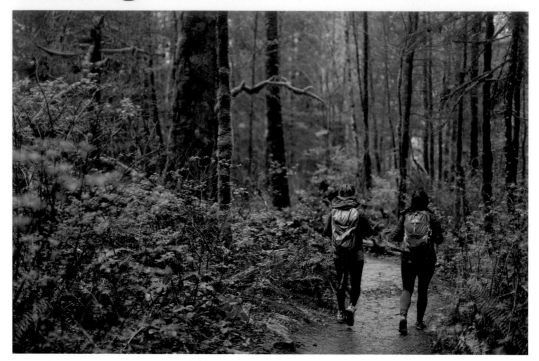

As a kid who grew up in the flat plains of suburban Chicago, I remember the first time I saw the red rock of Utah and went on my first hike. The combination of physical intensity, sweeping vistas, and immense skies became a steadying, driving force in my life.

By high school I'd discovered that hiking is my body's favorite kind of physical medicine, challenging me with tough trudges up steep slopes, pushing me to see where I need to strengthen my legs or glutes or feet, and forcing me to keep moving past obstacles like blisters or tired legs. It is mental medicine, too, a zone where my phone doesn't work, where my focus leaves email and to-do lists behind to navigate bulging tree roots and sharp rocks or to take in a peeka-boo view. From the sweeping green vistas in the rolling mountains of New Hampshire to the craggy peaks of Alaska, I have chosen schools and jobs so I can hike. It is my favorite way to move.

While hiking is akin to walking, when you add in elevation gain and exposure to temperature change, wind, sun, and more over several hours at a time, it becomes a major conditioning challenge for your body. You push your cardiovascular system, challenge your strength from legs to core and even your shoulders, and improve your balance over uneven terrain. Research suggests that being in nature eases stress levels, which can lower high blood pressure and risk of heart disease.

The simple fact is that hiking also takes you to places so miraculous, you can hear your heart beat in your chest and you wonder how you lived your whole life before seeing that place for yourself.

Over the years, I've learned there are different ways to challenge myself with hiking. My favorite is to hike with those I'm closest to—my partner, my dog, my dear friends—enjoying hours of easy conversation beyond daily tasks and logistics, discussing articles and books we've read recently, or simply walking in silence.

Occasionally, the challenge is to go with people I don't know. I took my first group hike with The Mountaineers, a Seattle-based nonprofit dedicated to helping people learn and conserve wild places in the Pacific Northwest and beyond. The Mountaineers organize many group hikes of varying difficulty, and I thought it would be fun to combine meeting new people with a favorite physical activity.

I chose a moderate pace option with a late afternoon start. I wanted an energetic, but not too intense, hike. It sounded like the ideal way to spend a summer evening. What I didn't know is that the after-hours hikers were renowned, to everyone but me, as fast hikers—they set a quick pace that means you

THE TEN ESSENTIALS

The point of the Ten Essentials, originated by The Mountaineers, has always been to answer two basic questions: Can you prevent emergencies and respond positively should one occur? And can you safely spend a night—or more—outside? Use this list as a guide and tailor it to the needs of your outing.

1. Navigation (map, altimeter, compass, GPS)
2. Headlamp
3. Sun protection (sunglasses, clothes, sunscreen, hat)
4. First aid
5. Knife
6. Fire (matches, lighter, and tinder)
7. Shelter (a light emergency blanket or tarp works)
8. Extra food
9. Extra water (or a purifier)
10. Extra clothes

could talk but it might be better for you to focus on getting enough oxygen to get up the mountain. If I had known, I might have been more prepared for a vigorous adventure. Hike and learn.

I showed up at the meeting place for a hike up Dirty Harry's Peak outside Seattle. The other six hikers were clearly experienced, avid members of The Mountaineers, including other hiking leaders. This was my first sign that my moderate hike might be more intense than I'd thought.

I usually like to hike with one or two people to get away from crowds. It was reassuring, however, to be in a larger group with leaders and a sweep at the rear to track everyone, oversee safety, and make sure we had the Ten Essentials (see sidebar). I also liked that someone else had chosen the route and would make sure we were on the right trail.

At the trailhead, I did my usual prep to get ready: tying my laces, putting on enough warm layers, and making sure I had everything set in my backpack, with easy access to water and snacks. I wasn't sure if we were going to stop much, and I wanted to be able to munch while hiking.

Once we were off, the group fell silent. It was a beautiful trail, and the woods soon filled with the steady sound of boots on dirt, poles thwacking rocks, and heavy breathing. I love quiet moments while hiking, but I was

HIKE IN MINIMAL SHOES

Some of the most challenging hiking terrain I ever encountered was the time I switched out of hiking boots to minimal shoes. Yes, I left the big, clunky boots behind.

I spent three months getting my feet ready to hike 6.5 miles and climb 1,900 feet or so in elevation. For 12 weeks, I stretched my feet using a half-dome roller and squishy balls to increase blood flow into my calves, Achilles, and feet. I walked barefoot over rocks outside my house. I switched out of tight, rigid, heeled shoes to flexible, flat ones. I walked on soft grass.

I was on a mission. I had read Katy Bowman's book *Whole Body Barefoot* and realized that a lifetime of wearing stiff-soled, heeled shoes while walking on flat, hard surfaces had created tight, inflexible feet. My stiff feet had a ripple effect up my body, affecting my knees, hips, lower back, and shoulders.

Before I could hike in minimal shoes, I had to train my feet. I wore minimal trail runners daily, marveling over every crack I could feel in the sidewalk. I rolled out aching feet at night. For my first hikes, I started in minimal shoes and carried trail runners with cushioned bottoms. When my feet felt tired and sore, I swapped them out.

After a few hikes, my feet were ready for that 6.5-mile hike. I was anxious—and determined.

The trail started with steep switchbacks. I felt the roots and uneven dirt under my feet, and I hiked more slowly to adjust. I made it to the top of the hike without much foot fuss. My feet felt good, and I was proud.

Coming back down, I was less jubilant. My knees often hurt on the way down, and they still did on this hike. Walking softly didn't alleviate the pain. Descending without limping felt like a win.

But I stuck with minimal shoes for daily wear and hiking, and over time, my knee pain disappeared altogether when hiking. By the next summer, I returned to my normal speedy hiking pace, hustling on the downhill with no pain in my feet or my knees, and I got rid of my trail runners.

I love how strong my feet are now, capable of walking over rocks without making me wince, and I am committed to keeping them that way.

accustomed to filtering through conversation topics first and then silence after everyone had tired, usually on the way down the mountain. Perhaps all the talking my friends and I do on a hike slows us down, I thought. Talk less, I reasoned, and you can go faster. In this case, that was true; we hiked at a good clip, faster than I usually start out. Twenty minutes in, I was covered in a sweaty sheen.

Our leader, Bill, acknowledged the pace was faster than the typical "moderate" pace, a technical level used by The Mountaineers in their hike ratings. But he looked us over and decided the group was strong and could handle it. Since we only had about a mile and a half to two miles of uphill on the five-mile hike, Bill kept the pace up while watching us. He would slow down if anyone looked like they needed it, he said.

I noticed that the familiar burn in my legs came on quickly on this hike; the trail gained about 1,300 feet in about two miles. A short, steep trail can be as difficult as a long one with gentler elevation gain. If the trail is hitting 1,000 feet of elevation in one mile, you're in for a steep hike. This one was, in other words, a decent amount of elevation gain.

We made quick time up the trail, taking a couple of breaks for water and to catch our breath. We slowed once we headed off toward Dirty Harry's Museum, which required some bushwhacking. Some folks had been there before, and I was happy to push through trees behind them as they looked for the "museum," a rusted logging truck abandoned by a man named Harry. After we crawled through trees that had grown around the truck and took a few pictures, we set off for Dirty Harry's Balcony, which offers majestic views of mountains to the south.

Bill was our guide and timekeeper, tracking our snack break at the top, as well as our head counter, making sure everyone stayed together. Basically, he kept us all in one piece, and it was awfully nice to have him around.

With a 4:30 p.m. start, we made it back to the trailhead before dark.

Being out with The Mountaineers, I saw my own habits around hiking with fresh eyes, including that I can broaden my hiking groups and pick up my pace. The leaders also gave a good reminder for how important it is to carry a good trail map for safety purposes. Going with a new group helped me see I was in a rut. Hiking can be more than a catch-up with friends or a quest for beautiful views; it can also be a time to explore a new trail, relax in the safety of a larger group, and meet kind people who love the same activity that you do.

I've hiked enough now to know that it doesn't matter if I hike with one person or a group; if I choose an intense, steep trail or a gentle one; or if my aim is to revel in a spectacular desert landscape or walk through a rainforest. If I want to get grounded, move my body, and feel genuine joy, the most important steps are to clear my schedule, get out of the house, and go.

GET STARTED HIKING

Get a pair of hiking boots (break them in before any serious adventures), trail runners, or minimal trail shoes, if you have worked up to minimal hiking (see sidebar). Do some research on local trails to see if you need any permits. Start with an easy three to four miles with 500 to 1,000 feet of elevation gain. Commit to hiking twice this month.

BEFORE YOU GO

Equipment: Hiking boots or trail runners with a good sole to handle rocks, slippery roots, and scree fields. Trekking poles (optional), waterproof layers, wool socks, and a backpack for carrying the Ten Essentials are an investment up front but will last for years.

Cost: Check fees for local trail access, trailhead parking passes, and park entrance; most one-day fees are $10 or less, but season passes may also be available.

CHALLENGE YOURSELF

Adding miles or elevation is all you need to ramp up the hiking challenge. Please note that the longer your hike, the more food and water you'll need to carry. After a couple of shorter hikes, push yourself with these goals:

Level Up: Head out for a longer hike of five to seven miles with elevation gain of 2,000 feet or so. The elevation makes a significant difference in the experience.

Reach Goal: Take on a longer hike of 8 to 10 miles, with 3,000 feet of elevation gain or more if you're feeling bold! Be mindful that this level of hike requires you to be in strong hiking condition, so be sure you've worked up to it with two or three five- to seven-mile hikes with steeper elevation before you head out. Also, make sure you have the Ten Essentials with you, and hike with one or two people for safety. Let others know where you're going and when you plan to be back.

Adventure Goal: Add in inflatable packrafts if you're headed to an alpine lake. The additional weight is worth the extra fun.

QUICK TIPS

- Trekking poles are helpful if you have knee pain. Downhill can be brutal on tender knees. Look into minimal shoes (see sidebar), which can help alleviate knee pain, though it takes time.
- Pack a real lunch. In my youthful 20s, I'd rush my way up mountains, eat a bar at the top, then fly back down. Now, my attitude is if I'm going to spend that much time getting to the view, I want to enjoy myself. I pack a full lunch and take my time at the top.
- Keep extra water, a change of shoes, and extra clothes in the trunk of your car. You'll be thirsty when you're done, and sweaty, and your feet will be tired.
- Don't wear cotton. You need clothes that wick away the sweat, because you will surely sweat, and they also need to keep you warm. Wear only synthetics or wool on the trail.
- Read recent trail reports online and check with relevant land managers before heading out. It's important to know if a road has been washed out, if the snowpack on a trail hasn't melted yet, or if there's snow higher up on your route.
- Check the weather and gear up appropriately for the conditions. Weather on a mountain can be significantly different from your weather at home and can turn fast, so it's best to be prepared.

DISCOVERY: *Hiking*

	1ST	2ND	3RD
DATE			
DURATION			
RATING (1 TO 5 STARS)	★ ★ ★ ★ ★	★ ★ ★ ★ ★	★ ★ ★ ★ ★

How did you feel the first time you went on a hike? What did you experience when you were outside and made it to your hike destination? What did you see, and what did you feel?

What did you learn about your own conditioning after your first more challenging hike?

What did you learn about the shift in mental state you experience from the beginning of a hike to how you feel at the end?

What was the most challenging part of the hike? What part did you find the most fulfilling? What surprised you about being on a hike?

Month **3**

Trampoline Jumping

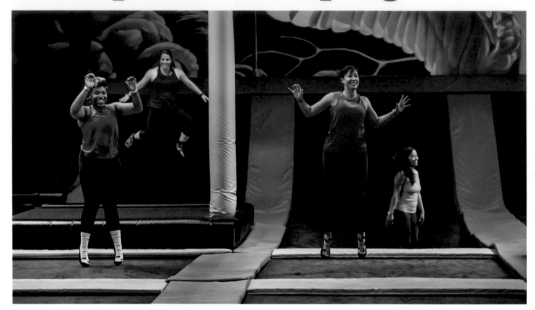

Thirty minutes? That's it? It was my first time at a trampoline play area, a giant warehouse space devoted to bouncing and usually filled with children bending the rule for only one jumper per trampoline.

I hadn't bounced since I was a kid, when my parents bought a mini-trampoline, which I jumped on while watching television. A 30-minute session struck me as a short—nay, even wimpy—amount of time to bounce, but a friend more experienced than I said it would be plenty. I agreed not to push it, though I secretly scoffed at the idea that trampolining would be much of a workout.

I was so innocent. Four days later, with my low back still feeling the effects of bouncing and my quads yelping with every move, my opinion of trampolining as a sport had radically changed.

The benefits of bouncing on a trampoline extend beyond sore quads and core; you also improve coordination and clarity and get an intense cardiovascular workout. Also, a word to the wise, particularly if you have lower back or knee pain: go easy at the beginning. Don't take your jumping up to the most intense level right away until you see how it feels; it is a high-impact activity, particularly on the bigger trampolines at a trampoline play center.

Bouncing on trampolines can be as much fun for adults as it is for kids. Jump up and down as high as you can go, throw yourself into the big foam pit, or head into the dodgeball arena if you feel aggressive and want to spike the ball. Since I would rather not be stung by an overzealous throw, probably chucked by an adult, I skip the dodgeball court, but it might be perfect for you.

Trampoline places are typically laid out in grids with a strict one-person-per-square rule that is enforced, but kids ignore anyway. There may be basketball hoops to practice jumping and dunking a ball or foam pits where you can learn to bounce, flip, or twist into a pit, gymnastics style.

After you have warmed up, the first, most important, most exciting thing to do is to get some air. If your body has given you the go-ahead, bounce as high as possible. I did that first; my hot tip is to windmill your arms to gain momentum. Go airborne as you jump higher and higher, your gaze floating out and above the trampoline walls. Your cheeks may stretch from smiling.

Next, I practiced jumping from tramp to tramp, bounding over the dividers separating the squares. It takes some momentum and practice to achieve one bounce per trampoline square—plus some skillful avoidance of kids trying to do the same thing or not paying attention whatsoever—but you'll soon be soaring across three, four, or five tramps at a time.

I did all of the above, loving the freedom of every bounce mixed in with nervousness that I might wipe out at any moment. Ten minutes in, I was dripping sweat, panting, and taking a break in front of a giant fan to cool off and catch my breath.

Jumping into the foam pit, filled with colorful, squishy cubes to cushion your landing, sounded like a break from the nonstop cardio. Inspired by Olympic gymnasts and divers, I bounced one square at a time toward the pit and flung myself rather awkwardly into the spongy blue, red, and yellow blocks. Once I mastered building bouncing momentum for more air time, I worked on a forward flip. I jumped in a big arc, reached for my feet with my hands to fold in half in the air and whipped my legs over my head so I landed upright. It took a few tries to land standing up instead of on my back, but once I focused on flinging my legs faster overhead, I started to land on my feet. Maybe those gymnastics lessons as a kid were paying off.

After I cooled down, I returned to the main trampoline and played with the diagonal walls on the tramp grids. I bounced across several squares, working up my momentum, then jumped up onto a diagonal wall tramp, turned around toward the regular squares, and tried to land on my feet in one. Landing on your feet is for cats, I decided, since I often fell. It seemed safer to work on tricks, and I practiced dropping on my rear and hopping back up to stand.

Did I mention that my legs were trembling? During the last few minutes of my half hour, I noticed my back and core were tired and sore. I was surprised they felt worn out, but at the time I was more concerned with mastering the perfect arc into the foam pit.

Thirty minutes flew by. By the time I left, I was scheming about the next time I could go bouncing.

Then the next day arrived. My lower back and abs were sore to a depth I hadn't felt in years; it was hard to do simple things like twist. My quads quivered with pain, and I limped on stairs. I had no idea how physically intense jumping for 30 minutes would be. I also realized my core and my legs were not as strong as I'd thought. My respect for Olympic gymnasts ballooned tenfold.

For the next week, I told everyone I had found the most killer workout ever. I don't think most believed me. Since then, I've become a trampoline devotee. I love to go to a trampoline park and bounce, though I'm better these days about pacing myself and not going crazy, especially since, if kids are involved, we stay for an hour.

Bouncing is exhilarating for everyone. There's nothing like the thrill of jumping higher than you thought you could, bounding from square to square, mastering new tricks, and grinning foolishly all the while. If you're a parent, you get an amazing workout while your kids play. I can't imagine a better family combo.

But what if you can't always get to a trampoline park, or perhaps there isn't one in your area? Though a mini-trampoline doesn't give the sensation of flying, it provides its own effective workout.

I had a mini at home as a kid. I think my mom sometimes used it for workout videos; I occasionally jumped on it but grew bored with it after the first few weeks. Today, mini-trampolines are still in use, and working out on them has a name—rebounding. A friend told me I needed to try it again and loaned me hers for a whirl at home.

While there is one famous study about the benefits of rebounding, those benefits have been disputed. I decided that rather than worrying about the accuracy of the science, I would bounce. I looked up some workouts on my friend Google and found a few different techniques for working out on my own at home. I pulled out the mini and got going, and I found I liked the simplicity and ease of bouncing at home.

I bounced for a couple of minutes to warm up, then started with some shoulder warm-ups, lifting my arms to the front and to the side. Many of the workouts recommend using small hand weights, which I didn't have, though they would increase the intensity and conditioning.

After the warm-up, I added in twists, which made bouncing on a small trampoline in my living room more fun. You swivel your torso while jumping, and the added effort works your entire core. If you keep your arms elevated, your shoulders will feel some extra intensity and strengthening.

The workout recommended straight up-and-down bouncing to work on form and to keep your core engaged. While it was challenging, I got bored. I longed for the bigger bounce from the larger trampoline squares at trampoline parks, and the major air time I could get there versus on the mini. To mix things up, I added in jumping jacks—and had to figure out coordinating my feet.

It's recommended that you do each exercise for 30 to 60 seconds. While 30 seconds wasn't long enough at the beginning, by the third or fourth exercise, I was winded. I sat down for crunches on the trampoline, rocking back and forth and using the bounce to add in core strengthening.

My favorite exercise was high knees, where you run in place, lifting your knees high to your chest and resisting the trampoline to make it harder. This one got my heart rate up immediately, and after 30 seconds, I took a break.

After just 10 minutes of rebounding exercises, my blood was pumping, and I felt reinvigorated after a morning in front of a computer.

My impatient side knows I'm not likely to rebound for more than 10 minutes at a time. I used a timer to keep myself going, but my mind still wandered. My ideal scenario would be to watch television and bounce for 10 to 15 minutes, likely at the end of the day if I needed to squeeze in more movement.

But you may be more disciplined than I am. If you have the tenacity to bounce for 20 to 25 minutes, you'll work up a big sweat and feel the impact. My legs and core tired out quickly when I pushed myself on the mini-trampoline. And I know any activity is better than none.

If a mini-trampoline—or any trampoline at all—is calling your name, go for it. Find out why the kids are having so much fun.

GET STARTED TRAMPOLINING

Go to a trampoline park and book 30 minutes. Go easy on yourself and take breaks when you need to, particularly if you have not jumped before. If you're working on a mini-tramp, jump for 10 to 15 minutes.

QUICK TIPS

- Wear clothes fit for sweating. You'll work your entire body, and you'll get sweaty fast.
- Start out bouncing gently, warming up and seeing how your body handles bouncing. Build your endurance and take a lot of breaks; jumping for even one minute solid will kick your heart rate up right away.

BEFORE YOU GO

Equipment: Shoes, though you also can bounce barefoot. Some trampoline places require socks with grips on the soles.

Cost: Most trampoline play areas charge by the amount of time you jump, generally starting with an hour. An hour typically costs $15 to $20.

CHALLENGE YOURSELF

Start slowly. It's easy to ramp up intensity by bouncing higher and for longer stretches of time. After you've done your first 30-minute session, add to the fun in these ways:

Level Up: Go to a trampoline park for a 30-minute session again and see if you can jump for longer stretches between breaks and increase your endurance. Challenge yourself with some jumps into the foam pit. For a mini-tramp, increase your frequency to twice a week for 10- to 15-minute sessions.

Reach Goal: Increase your time at a trampoline park to 60 minutes. Push yourself to bounce for even longer periods of time or boldly enter the dodgeball court. For a mini-tramp, see if you can increase your time to 20 to 25 minutes and do it three times a week.

Adventure Goal: Check out classes on wall trampolines, learning more tricks, or other offerings. Watch online videos to find new tricks you can practice at the park.

DISCOVERY: *Trampoline Jumping*

	1ST	2ND	3RD
DATE			
DURATION			
RATING (1 TO 5 STARS)	★ ★ ★ ★ ★	★ ★ ★ ★ ★	★ ★ ★ ★ ★

Did you resist the idea of bouncing on a trampoline, thinking it's just for kids? How did you feel when you started bouncing?

I pooh-poohed the idea that jumping on a trampoline required strength. What did you discover about your strength or areas that jumping would help you strengthen?

What did you learn about moving your body on a trampoline?

How did you feel at the end of the session? Were you happier? Did you have fun?

RECOVERY: *Massage*

There was a time I associated massage with relaxation. I liked the calming music, the low light, the little nap on the massage table.

Nowadays, my massages come with gritted teeth and deep breathing, waiting for the intense, uncomfortable sensations shooting up my forearm or through my shoulder to pass. While there is some soothing music playing in the background, I don't feel all that calm. I telepathically send SOS signals to my therapist: Please hurry.

I push my body, and as a result, things can hurt or feel off. An old hip injury and a recurring shoulder injury have prompted me to see a professional bodywork practitioner for help in recovery and healing. In my experience, massage is most useful when your therapist takes a healing approach, identifying unhealthy movement patterns and helping with recovery.

I began working with Sam Hammer, an orthopedic massage therapist who focuses on structural integration massage, working on connective tissue, with a physical therapy approach. Hammer works with active people who like high-intensity workouts or weight lifting, and people with pain or alignment issues. He assesses movement patterns first. If you're active, you're more likely to notice if something is off because you feel it in your sport or training, he said. Older folks can also benefit from basic movement training for flexibility to prevent future injury, help keep arthritis at bay, or understand how a limited range of motion affects balance and strength. Hammer looks at the root cause of mis-alignment and works on the core issue and the current area of pain and injury.

My shoulder hurt from years of carrying a heavy purse, and the pain flared in yoga classes. Over time it went away; then it showed up again after I did kipping pull-ups (swinging and using my legs and a hip snap to pull my chin up over a bar). When I took a break from kipping and rested my shoulder, it got better, but I kept injuring it again. I wanted it resolved, if that was possible.

After watching me move, Hammer noted that one of the biggest issues was tightness in my biceps and forearms from repetitive movement typing on the computer. Did he say this to a writer?

My mid-back also was stiff due to sitting, which meant I wasn't twisting effectively. Did he say this to a yoga teacher?

As Hammer started working my forearms and biceps, I grimaced. My fascia was twisted in my shoulder area, pulling it out of optimal alignment. Side note: None of us have opti-mal alignment for reasons related to how we use our bodies. Essentially, all of us have adapted movement patterns, whether from a lack of movement or previous injuries.

My tissue was responsive and healthy, a good sign for changing movement patterns, Hammer said. Thank heavens. Despite my funky shoulder and tight forearms, all the ways I love to move have done the job of keeping my body healthy, strong, and mobile.

Hammer worked my shoulder, and I felt it soften as he pushed into the areas that hurt the most. He told me to breathe while he worked my mid-back and helped me rotate more. Tightness in my mid-back was potentially causing me to over-rotate through my shoulders, creating pain. It also was an issue that led to other problems (see "Recovery: Healing from Injury" in Month 6).

Hammer looked at my feet. I rely too heavily on my toes to flex my feet, instead of using my ankles. He noted tightness in my shins, which kept me from using my ankles. Runners with ankles that overpronate in or supinate out often have tightness in their joints or shins that, once released, can change how they run.

Was there any area of my body that wasn't tight?

Hammer gave me an exercise to release tightness in my forearms from typing, and another to support twisting from my mid-back to build new movement patterns into my body.

Almost everyone has movement patterns to work on. It's wise for athletes to have their movement patterns assessed before taking on major physical challenges, such as running a marathon or lifting heavy weights, which can exaggerate unhealthy patterns. Even tightness in your hips in your 40s or 50s can lead to arthritic hips and the need for hip replacements later. Shifting unhealthy movement patterns as soon as possible makes a difference.

Hammer's assessment deepened my respect for how complicated the body is and how essential it is to work with someone who has studied the body and techniques for keeping it healthy and strong.

I once thought of massage as a way to relax. Now I see it as a way to support my body so I can stay active, strong, and mobile.

Tennis

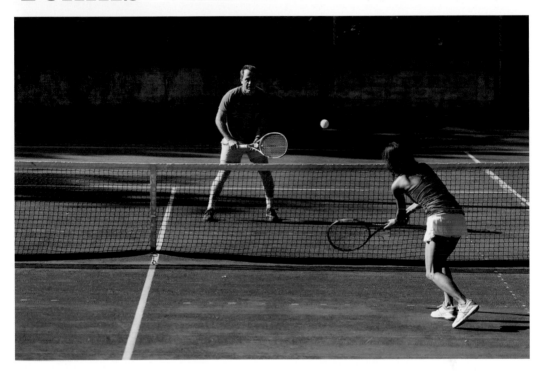

In high school, I played a lot of tennis, competing in doubles against other high school teams in the fall and training in the summer with competitive singles matches on midwestern courts that radiated heat while I ran after forehands and backhands. I loved tennis. I loved the camaraderie of heading out with a friend to train and the thrill of an amazing smash or a winning backhand.

When I went to college, I pretty much left tennis behind. I rarely looked back, aside from a few pickup games with friends, where I joyfully rallied from the baseline and hit hard ground strokes, happy I still had the muscle know-how to do so.

Fast-forward a couple decades, when some of my tennis-playing friends discovered I had secret skills. They considered my self-imposed exile a travesty. They bugged me to join an adult tennis league and re-hone my teenage abilities. They told me how much fun it was. While my competitive spirit was alive

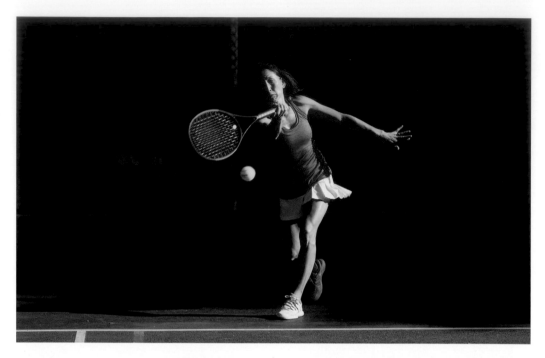

in workouts, going into a tennis league felt like too much of a commitment. I begged off with the original excuse: "I'm too busy."

Of course, I wondered what it would be like to serve, return, and hit hard again. I wondered if I was any good. I'd spent so much time on a tennis court in high school, it seemed a shame to let all that effort and time spent practicing and going to weekend tournaments as a teenager go to waste. So I decided to take a lesson and find out if my tennis spirit lived on.

Many people play tennis well into their golden years for good reason. Beyond the fact that the sport is low-impact, studies have found that tennis players tend to have better aerobic and cardiovascular fitness. They also have better bone health, even if they start playing as an adult, not to mention developing and then maintaining hand-eye coordination.

I headed out to meet Kate, a pro at a local tennis club. Equipment technology has changed quite a bit in the 20 years since I last bought a racket, so she picked out a few rackets for me to try, and then we headed to a court to warm up.

After rallying with me for a few rounds and watching my technique, Kate asked if I wanted to play a game or if I wanted to learn the "new style" of tennis. New style? I was perplexed. To me, a forehand was a forehand. How could that have changed in the last two decades?

I was so, so wrong.

So many components of tennis have changed, starting with the technology for tennis rackets. I thought rackets were light in high school, but they've gotten even tougher and lighter in the years since I left the game. As a result, technique shifted to preserve power and speed.

Kate looked at my grip first, moving it from continental (with my thumb wrapped around the bottom of the handle) to a semi-western (with my hand positioned a quarter turn back around the racket). Instead of my usual big windup, ready to blast a tennis ball across the court, Kate showed me how to loop my racket back and down like a Ferris wheel. After I hit the ball, I swung my racket across my body and caught it with my left hand like a pizza tray at shoulder height. The first couple of times I did it, I had no power—and no control, to boot. But then it started to land right, and I could see that this loop creates more spin and control, even if it felt awkward at first.

The baseline setup position had also changed. I once held the racket low in front of me, ready for a forehand or a backhand. Think of a pro player in an alert, ready position. Most players now hold their rackets upright in front of their chests as they run across the court, ready to hit the ball with a massive amount of topspin.

Lastly, Kate told me to stop flipping my head up along with my racket whenever I hit the ball and instead keep it level and still through the stroke.

All of the changes felt uncomfortable and, frankly, wrong. The grip bugged me the most. I wanted to move my hand back to my old hand position and hit hard the way I had

OR TRY . . . SQUASH

I knew the geometry of squash and mastering the angles of an indoor court would be tough. In truth, I should have prepared for relentless sprinting.

My teacher, Shabana, said the squash racket is like a cousin to the tennis racket, which explained why I am more at home with squash than indoor racket sports like racquetball. But there are differences—courts with boundary lines on the walls and a ball with almost no bounce. I spent a lot of time chasing that tiny, not-so-bouncy ball.

Shabana started me with a rally. I forgot to hustle to the ball, which dies in a flash. I questioned if I was fast enough as I whiffed. I also swung at the ball tennis style and had to learn the squash technique—extend your arm, keep the racket parallel to the ground. If I stretched my arm for my follow-through, I hit well.

To ramp things up, I hit 10 shots in a row. My legs burned, and I was breathless from chasing the ball. Next, I practiced hitting down the line. Placement forces opponents into a corner, Shabana said. I struggled to return deep corner shots. Slow down your swing, and be patient, she said.

Finally, she asked if I wanted a break. Phew. Yes, please. I looked at the clock. Only 22 minutes in, I was sweaty and panting.

After the break, we played some full points. Shabana's masterful placement ran me all over the court. I tried to hit closer to the wall to force her to run. She applauded my intention, though she still won pretty much every point.

By the end of my lesson, I was ready to pass out. But I loved it. If I had regular access to a squash court, I would be back, chasing that seriously not-bouncy ball.

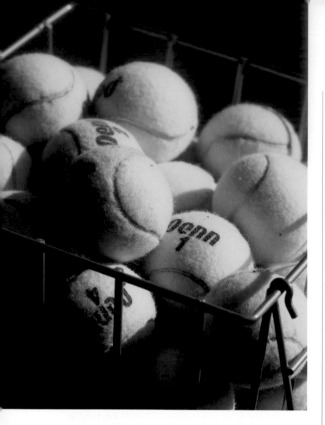

originally learned. The first couple of times I hit a forehand, my ball went right where I predicted—straight into the net. I was frustrated. Kate was patient. She repeated, "Set, Ferris wheel, and pizza tray." Set my racket in the upright position, loop it in a Ferris wheel, finish in a pizza tray position on my opposite shoulder, and catch the racket with my left hand. So. Many. Cues.

Kate tossed me ball after ball until I understood the looping motion. I started to get the ball across the net and saw more extreme topspin with an impressively high bounce on the other side of the court. I stopped trying to hit hard and worked on technique.

Once I hit the ball over the net consistently, and it got closer to the baseline instead of coming up short, Kate looked at my footwork. The new upright racket setup confused me, and I had compensated with a weird shuffle

toward the ball instead of a jog. Running to the ball rather than shuffling, while holding my racket upright in the new position, required more coordination than I expected. I had to practice.

But slowly, the pieces came together. I could tell when I hit well with the new technique. I was delighted when my topspin worked and the ball landed with a huge bounce on the other side. Kate reminded me to hold my racket higher and stop shuffling.

Once I got a sense of how to execute the forehand every time and felt comfortable with the technique, we moved to the backhand. I learned that it also had evolved since I last played regularly. I wanted to throw a tennis tantrum and hurl my racket. As with the forehand, Kate showed me how to move my grip to a semi-western position when I ran to hit backhand so that my left hand was in a position to create the same looping swing.

Running toward a backhand with my racket in the new, higher position, I quickly switched my hand from the forehand to backhand grip (in my old style—they stayed almost the same), another layer of challenge for my already tired brain. We were messing with my favorite stroke, and I was in a mini-revolt. With a lot of practice hitting easy tosses, I started to pick this one up, too, though it didn't feel natural.

I love the physical challenge of teaching my body to move in new ways. In some respects, the return to a familiar sport while weaving in a new approach made tennis adventurous again. Learning the new techniques reminded me of all the drills I'd done as a teenager. I also relished being around the rubbery smell of tennis balls and the resonant thwack of ball against tennis strings when the ball hits the sweet spot. I remembered the power and speed of the game.

As much fun as I had, I needed more practice to cement the new style and stop hitting the ball into the net before I could play a game. Kate and I didn't work on my serve, but I'm sure it needs major resuscitation, like the rest of my tennis game. As for joining a tennis league, well, that's a commitment I haven't been willing to step into. A few more tennis lessons are in order first.

GET STARTED PLAYING TENNIS

If you've never played before, take a private lesson at a club or a community center and learn some basic skills, and then join some pickup games with others at your level. If you've played before, head out with a friend to hit on a court and see how it feels to get back in the groove. Play once a week and have fun.

BEFORE YOU GO

Equipment: Racket, tennis shoes, tennis balls. You can rent rackets at tennis clubs, which is useful if you want to try and eventually buy one that is a newer model.

Cost: Free outdoors; indoor court rental ranges in cost from $30 to $50, not including member fees for private tennis clubs.

QUICK TIPS

- If you learned tennis as a kid, be aware that some aspects of the game may have changed since then. Don't be afraid to take some lessons to brush up on your skills and learn new techniques.
- If you haven't played in a few years, consider investing in a new racket. Rackets are constantly being improved.
- Wear non-scuffing shoes, and bring fresh tennis balls that have good bounce.

CHALLENGE YOURSELF

Once you feel comfortable with technique, step up your game with these goals:

Level Up: If you're new, add in one additional practice time per week to hit the ball and work on technique. For experienced players, sign up for a private lesson and work on your form. Layer in some competition by keeping score and playing a full set.

Reach Goal: The challenge in tennis heats up once you add competition. For new players, keep score and play a full set with someone at a similar level. For experienced players, play a full match with someone else at a similar level.

Adventure Goal: Whether you're a newer player or an experienced one, join a league at your level and turn competitive tennis into a regular part of your life.

DISCOVERY: *Tennis*

	1ST	2ND	3RD
DATE			
DURATION			
RATING (1 TO 5 STARS)	★ ★ ★ ★ ★	★ ★ ★ ★ ★	★ ★ ★ ★ ★

If tennis is new to you, how did you feel the first time you hit a good, solid forehand or backhand? What did you learn about your hand-eye coordination and the challenge of learning a new sport?

What was it like the first time you kept score and added competition to your game? Were you motivated or frustrated when winning or losing points?

If you played when you were younger, what did you love about tennis back then? What is your goal now that you are returning to the sport?

What did you notice about muscle memory when you played again for the first time? Did playing come back easily, or was it difficult to play like you once did?

Month **4**

Tree Climbing

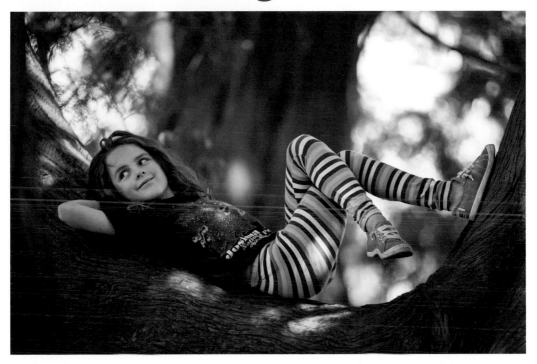

My approach to activity with kids is oriented around a few favorites—a trip to the pool, a playground, or a trampoline park. Kids also love to climb trees. When I have my stepkids, we'll head to our favorite park, where we make our way to a cluster of old trees with long, graceful limbs. Once there, we easily spend an hour climbing and crawling around.

If you have kids, you may find you can't keep them out of trees. Climbing a tree is one of the original ways humans moved through the world—to gather fruit, to see farther, to find shelter. Today, it's a movement activity you can do anywhere there are trees, and at any age.

When I found out that Rafe Kelley, founder of Evolve Move Play, makes room for kids in his outdoor movement classes, I was excited about a structured way for adults and kids to move together—and get better at climbing trees. Rafe teaches a form of natural movement with roots in parkour, and I knew his approach would include time in trees, the real reason my tree-loving stepkids, Reagan and Carson, wanted to go.

Tree climbing provides benefits beyond balance; climbing a tree can also improve cognitive skills including memory, because it requires you to calculate and evaluate spatial awareness, balance, and orientation. One study found that after two hours of climbing, people's working memory had improved by 50 percent. Basically, your brain is on high alert after climbing a tree.

For class, we met at a local park in Seattle, where adults and kids gathered in a circle to warm up; Carson and Reagan made faces at each other. Rafe took us through wrist and shoulder warm-ups. For our necks, he told the kids to move like a snake side to side and bob their heads forward like a dolphin. They complied, sort of.

We headed to a nearby cluster of trees with long, thick branches and bark worn smooth from thousands of climbers. Rafe showed us our first challenge—walk up wide, low tree branches without using hands. He demonstrated the route, walking smoothly up the tree and going several branches higher than my comfort zone, especially with only hard ground down below.

Rafe made it look simple. Once my turn came, I realized how hard it was to stay balanced. During the first round, everyone was

OR TRY . . . PARKOUR

I knew I was in trouble when my fit parkour teacher, Ben, told us he loved parkour because something always scares him.

Parkour is the art of forward movement, moving on or around obstacles, usually outside on buildings or in the street. It's inspiring. Until you do it. When Ben told us the day's theme—"high to low"—I visualized crazy flips from a tall wall to the floor at the indoor parkour gym. Heights are part of parkour. I wondered if they should have a test at the front door for scaredy-cats.

After warm-ups, we practiced cushioning ourselves on falls. We went to a big platform, hopped up, and practiced exits, from a straight hop down to a reverse spin and a parkour roll, similar to a somersault.

For a wall step, we ran toward a wall, stepped one foot on the wall, jumped up, and landed softly to practice the explosive energy required to grab and get up on top of a wall. I was certain I was too short. Ben watched me and said, "You can reach the top. You just have to believe you can."

Yes, they practice Jedi mind tricks on you in parkour.

For "skin the cat," I reached for a pull-up bar, pulled my legs to my chest, and spun my legs through my arms to hang down behind me. I looped one leg over the bar to whip myself up to a sitting position. This, I could do.

If you loved playing on a jungle gym as a kid, you will be at home in parkour. I used every muscle in my body to hang from bars, jump, and somersault. I'd do it again, despite my nerves.

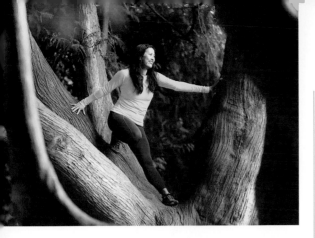

tentative, working out footing and wobbling along the route. Going from one thick tree branch to another without hands requires deep hip strength and trust in your footwear. With each round, everyone got more comfortable and made it up a little higher. I was impressed watching the kids try to get to higher branches.

After a few practice rounds, Rafe switched routes on the same tree. This route was low to the ground but had a bigger step up to a higher branch, requiring strong leg and glute action to get there. It was slightly easier to navigate, though I needed my hands get to the final branch. We practiced this route a few times to get the hang of a wiggly branch, but it was a little easier than the first one.

Next, we practiced jumping over and through branches. Rafe showed us an obstacle course on a dead tree that was trimmed down to several undulating branches low to the ground. Rafe had brought his kids to class and demonstrated the course over and around the branches with his then-almost-four-year-old son, who showed us a lower, easier route while Rafe demonstrated how to jump over the higher branches. They both made it look smooth and fun as they raced through the branches.

Then it was our turn. Adults and kids both went for it. The first jump on the adult route was relatively high, so I scrambled up onto the branch, then switched over to the lower kid route to make it easier. I liked watching experienced adults jump over branches, sometimes with a smooth leap, other times by putting one foot up and scrambling over. The kids climbed over the tall roots or ran underneath arcs in the wood. To increase the excitement and challenge, Rafe also had adults chase kids and vice versa; his four-year-old chased me, giggling with his arms stretched out.

While we waited our turn, Carson clambered into thinner nearby trees he called "koala" trees. Rafe climbed up there with him, telling him to swing as fast as he could to another small tree before Rafe, who had turned into a "tree shark," could get him. Carson sped up, reaching from branch to branch and weaving his way through.

When it was clear the kids' attention had wandered, Rafe's assistant teacher, Andrew, went to work with them on technique on a different tree.

The adults honed in on jumping over tree branches. When you jump over a branch, the goal is to keep momentum moving forward and land your feet in a running motion. Rafe also taught us a step vault—jumping with one leg up, pulling the other through, and putting your hands down on the tree branch to slide both feet to the ground, which makes it easier to keep running afterward. Eventually, he said, you can plant both hands on the branch and jump with both legs through at the same time. I never mastered that move, but my vaults got smoother. I could jump one foot up onto the branch, put my hands down, slide my other leg through and off the branch, and keep running.

Rafe closed down the class by gathering us all for a few deep breaths as a light rain began to fall. Despite a bee sting mid-class for Carson, the kids asked if they could climb trees again the next day.

On our second outing, everyone was bolder. We all were more willing to trust our feet to climb higher into the branches. Carson and Reagan showed me tic-tacs—running up to the tree, jumping their feet off the trunk, and landing on the ground—which they learned with Andrew. I love how kids intuitively want to climb trees, but so do adults.

When I'm in a tree, my relationship to the tree changes. I notice how strong its limbs are. I realize how deep the roots must be. I think about all the years it's been alive. I feel a kinship with the tree. When we're all out on a tree climbing adventure, I hang off branches to strengthen my arms. I try to climb higher than the last time I was there. Sometimes, I climb up onto a branch, settle into a perch, and watch kids swing and crawl around me.

GET STARTED TREE CLIMBING

Finding a good tree is the easiest way to start. Check out local parks and look up—you might see kids guiding you to your perfect climbing tree. Find a sturdy tree with low branches, and practice stepping up onto the lowest branch and feeling comfortable getting up into the tree.

BEFORE YOU GO

Equipment: Comfortable, flexible shoes with good grip on the sole.
Cost: Free.

CHALLENGE YOURSELF

Once you're comfortable on the low branches, reach new heights with these goals:

Level Up: Start to climb higher into branches. Choose one where you can sit for a moment and feel more comfortable about getting higher into the tree.
Reach Goal: Climb higher into the tree, staying close to the trunk. Make sure branches are sturdy!
Adventure Goal: Canopy climbing uses rock climbing equipment to scale 150-foot trees. See if there are guided canopy climbing opportunities in your area, and reach incredible heights in your tree climbing.

QUICK TIPS

- You need to use your feet to climb a tree well, even though your tendency will likely be to rely on your arms to pull yourself up. Practice stepping onto a branch with your feet and using your arms for stability rather than strength.
- Stay close to the trunk while climbing. That's where branches are strongest.
- Grab a branch and hang from it to strengthen and stretch your shoulders. Try swinging your legs up to wrap around the branch and hang that way. Climb frequently enough, and the skin on your hands also will get tougher.

DISCOVERY: *Tree Climbing*

	1ST	2ND	3RD
DATE			
DURATION			
RATING (1 TO 5 STARS)	★ ★ ★ ★ ★	★ ★ ★ ★ ★	★ ★ ★ ★ ★

What came up for you the first time you started climbing a tree? What did you notice about the tree? What did you notice about your response to being in a tree?

What was it like when you started to climb higher? Did you get nervous or feel anxious? Were you able to calm yourself down when you got up higher? How did you calm down?

How did you feel once you were in the tree for a while? Were you able to pause and look around? What did you see?

Stand-Up Paddleboarding

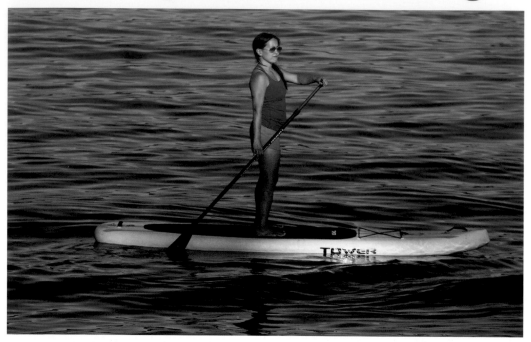

The first time I saw someone stand-up paddleboarding—let's be honest, it was probably a celebrity on the cover of a magazine—I thought it looked unstable and slow. I pooh-poohed it as a physical challenge. How could you get any kind of impact or strengthening from something that looked so, well, easy?

Then the word spread about stand-up paddleboarding, also known as SUP, and as more people did it, on all kinds of bodies of water from lakes to oceans, I knew it was time to stop judging so hard. I got on a board and went wobbling about on the water. I felt uncomfortable, like I was about to take a plunge at any moment.

Naturally, I fell in love.

I like paddle sports. I've played on river kayaks. I did a three-day river canoeing trip in college. I feel comfortable paddling on the water. But going from sitting to standing was a pronounced change. When you stand on a paddleboard, you can better use your core for power and fluidity, which elevates it above a

OR TRY . . . CANOEING

Whenever I want to be on the water with near-zero risk of getting wet, I canoe. You can also make it as hard or as relaxed as you like; some days I want the latter.

My friend Natalie and I met on a beautiful day at a place where canoe rentals are inexpensive and simple. Sign a waiver, get a life jacket and a paddle, and you're off in a metal canoe on Lake Washington, a large lake that divides the city of Seattle from the suburbs.

We felt unhurried. I was in charge of steering, and it took practice to keep us straight by holding my paddle close to the canoe or to turn the canoe by sticking my paddle into the water at an angle for a J-stroke. We zigzagged our way toward a slough, gliding over lily pads and past geese and ducks.

We hung close to shore, the stands of a nearby stadium dominating the horizon to our left, and the lake and a large bridge to our right. It was beautiful and quiet; it felt like we had the lake to ourselves. We paddled most of the hour and a half at a leisurely pace, peeping at lakefront homes. We even debated taking a swim, but it wasn't hot and we weren't dressed for it, so we continued paddling.

The return to the dock where we'd started took a little more effort—we had traveled farther than I thought. I was surprised to feel worn out by the end.

Canoeing is one of the simplest ways to enjoy being on the water and to move at your own pace. Rent a canoe, grab your paddle, put on your life jacket, and enjoy.

kayak or a canoe. I loved seeing farther, going faster, and getting in and out of the water more easily. It's also simple to hop off for a quick dip.

To be fair, that power comes with a lot of effort. Despite my early judgment that stand-up paddleboarding looked easy, it isn't. The boards aren't stable. Your core may be worn out after a stint on a stand-up paddleboard.

For most people, their first inclination on a paddleboard is to stay on their knees, where your center of gravity is lower and it feels more stable on the wobbly board. But staying on your knees doesn't give you as much leverage and power when executing a long stroke. The speed and strength are part of the fun and excitement of a paddleboard. Get the guts to stand up, and you'll immediately wonder

why you bothered with kneeling, even if you feel shaky on your feet and ponder how high the risk of slipping into the water is.

The first time I got on a paddleboard, my instructor told me to stand with my feet roughly hip-width distance on either side of the handle, knees slightly bent for balance. You keep your weight evenly on your feet. The stroke is simple, especially if you have experience with other paddle sports. Dip your blade into the water and trace the side of the board. The more you leverage the strength of your legs, torso, and shoulders for each stroke, the farther and faster you skim on the water.

Practicing control of your paddleboard is essential. If you've done any kind of paddling before, turning with a wide sweep stroke or hooking your blade into the water toward the back edge of the board to turn right or left quicker will come naturally. If not, it may take some practice to get used to your speed and an unsteady paddleboard. Once you get the hang of a paddleboard, it can be an idyllic way to spend a couple of hours.

It also can be a major cardiovascular challenge, especially if you decide to push yourself in, say, a race environment. No matter your experience level, being on a board on the water will test your core strength and improve your balance. An added benefit? It is low impact.

Let's get back to racing.

When I heard about people who raced paddleboards, I was intrigued, though I didn't feel like I had the skills to join them. I'm competitive by nature, but my competitiveness has limits. Racing in an activity I don't do

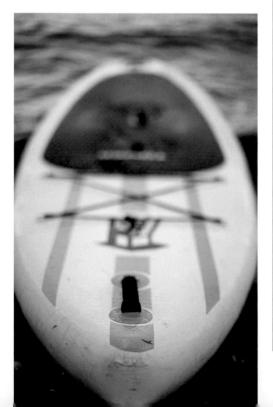

regularly is one of them, particularly when it involves frigid ocean water and the potential to fall in.

I asked the folks who organized a weekly race held at a local Elks club if I could observe and learn, and they welcomed me in. I was thrilled to learn there was a fun course for people like me—people who want to get out on the water but aren't interested in being timed or trying to compete with the group.

When race day arrived, I looked out the window and noted the constant wind gusting through the trees, blowing branches every which way. I had paddled enough to know that going straight into wind is not a good time; the risk of falling into the aforementioned chilly water goes up along with knot speed.

The organizers told me the fun course came with a guide, so someone would keep an eye on me in case anything happened. All racers also were required to carry a personal flotation device, or PFD, i.e., a life jacket.

The competitive racers gathered in the parking lot adjacent to the bay where they'd race. Jim, a longtime racer, loaned me his paddleboard and a PFD. The race was open to anyone with a board, paddle, and PFD; kayakers and other paddlers were welcome, though stand-up paddleboard was the most popular choice.

It was time to gear up. Despite the chilly evening, I noticed the other participants were wearing light layers; some wore only shorts and a long-sleeved shirt. I felt cautious about the windy conditions and accepted a loan of a wetsuit shirt and booties.

We all headed down to a sandy cove, where we listened to course instructions and paid attention to key landmarks to stay on track. Once the instructions were done, the competitive racers got into the water first, holding their boards and waiting for the signal to start. As soon as the whistle blew, there was a flurry of running and jumping onto boards and furious paddling to get out to the bay.

I hung back with my paddleboard guide, Joe, and watched the pack paddle off. Then Joe had me bring my board to the water and get on.

I tried to remember my paddling technique—soft knees, keeping the strokes short, and using my core to propel myself forward. I felt slow, especially compared to the racers. Even when I tried to go faster by paddling quicker or using a stronger stroke, I fell behind the competitive racers. I wasn't racing, and I still felt disgruntled at how far behind I was. I said I was competitive, okay?

Joe was in no rush. He gave me a couple tips as we moved out of the protected cove. I relaxed and looked out across the water at dramatic clouds skittering across the sky and the gray, bumpy water with a few whitecaps breaking farther out. I remembered how beautiful paddling is. I watched the racers hug the shore for a short stretch, then hurry off across the bay.

We followed the group at a leisurely pace, passing some other fun course participants who sat on their boards, legs hanging in the water and chatting as they watched the racers. They waved at us.

As we paddled out farther, Joe asked if I wanted to head into more open water, where the waves were rougher.

"Yes," I said out loud. Inside, I thought, Wait, is this a good idea?

To prep, he told me if a wave came over the front lip of the board to jump back slightly to counter the weight with my own. While his

tip was helpful, it wasn't encouraging; what if I fell when jumping back?

I remembered that the best way to paddle into rough wind and water is to aim the tip of my board into the waves; when you turn your board sideways or parallel to waves, that's when you can get knocked off. I also reminded myself that if I felt tense, my chances of falling also increased.

We paddled for a bit, and I tried not to grip my paddle for dear life. As my board rode up and down the cadence of the waves, I told myself to relax my shoulders. Finally, Joe asked if I wanted to turn back. I nodded, when I really wanted to shout, "*Yes, please.*"

Turning was tougher, and I tensed when I felt my board shift and get tippy as waves pushed against the length of the board. But Joe talked me through it, and I was able to steer myself back in the opposite direction and let the waves push us back toward the safety of the cove.

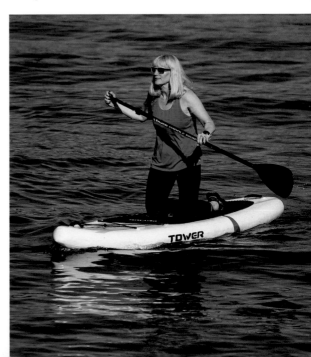

Once the wind was at our backs, paddling got more stable, and we moved a lot quicker. In the calmer water by the shore, I lifted my eyes, which had been glued to the waves and my board, to spot the racers. I could barely see a few of them, far beyond where we turned around.

I was amazed at their endurance and tenacity considering the weather. Joe said they were fighting harsh conditions.

Yeah, tell me about it.

We stayed at our leisurely pace paddling back to the beach where we'd started and waited for them to come in.

The fastest racer finished the course in about 25 minutes. I realized I wasn't the only one who struggled with the rough water. A few of them went the wrong way on the course. One racer commented, "I was getting hammered." Another called the bumps "fun."

To each their own.

Getting on a paddleboard might seem a solitary pursuit, but seeing the camaraderie among the competitive racers and those on the fun route reminded me that a communal passion and experience is all you need to connect with other people, no matter the activity. Paddle with others, and you're far more likely to test your limits. I know I did.

GET STARTED STAND-UP PADDLEBOARDING

Find a local paddleboard shop and take a lesson. Learn the foundations of paddleboarding with a group and get basic paddling technique down.

QUICK TIPS

- It can get chilly on the water, especially if you fall in! Bring some layers or check to see if you can rent a wet or dry suit.
- Start on your knees. Don't force yourself to stand up on a paddleboard until you're ready.

BEFORE YOU GO

Equipment: Paddleboard and paddle, available for rent. Rental places provide a PFD, and most have wet suits or dry suits if needed. Unless you plan to take a swim, shorts or workout leggings generally work.

Cost: The price of rentals varies depending on the place and the amount of time you have the paddleboard, typically $30 to $40 for two hours.

CHALLENGE YOURSELF

Once you're comfortable on the water, it likely won't take a lot of convincing for you to spend more time paddling. After a lesson, try these goals:

Level Up: Rent a board and go out for an hour. Challenge yourself to stay standing the whole time. Make sure you go with a paddling buddy.

Reach Goal: Take a paddleboard out for two hours or more and see what it feels like to paddle for an extended period of time. If you're really feeling ready, consider investing in your own paddleboard.

Adventure Goal: See if there is a local paddleboard race and join in the competition.

DISCOVERY: *Stand-Up Paddleboarding*

	1ST	2ND	3RD
DATE			
DURATION			
RATING (1 TO 5 STARS)	★ ★ ★ ★ ★	★ ★ ★ ★ ★	★ ★ ★ ★ ★

How did you feel the first time you went out on the water? Did you feel comfortable or were you nervous about getting on a paddleboard?

What did you learn about your relationship to water and how you feel about it?

What did you experience physically while paddling? Were you surprised by anything about your own conditioning from your time on the water?

What was your favorite part of paddling? What was your biggest challenge?

Month 5

Yoga

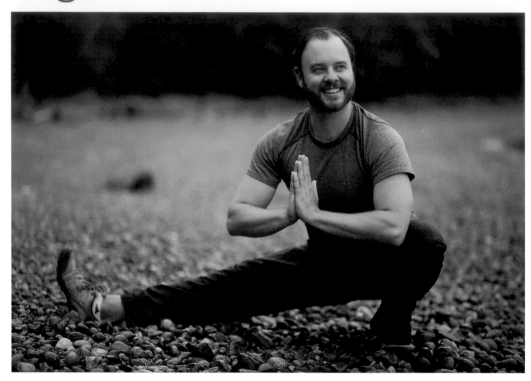

I was bent over at the waist, reaching my hands toward the ground in a wide-legged forward fold. Sweat dripped off my nose. I felt cocooned, swaddled in warmth and sweat. My legs also trembled from the effort. I wondered when class would be over.

I was at my first-ever power yoga class, and while I thought I had done a decent number of yoga classes up until that point, I had never sweated quite like this. I didn't recall

sweating as much ever in my life, or at least that's how my dramatic side felt. My hands slipped in downward-facing dog on my mat. (I made a mental note to get a better towel.) During tree pose, my foot was so sweaty, it slid down my leg. (I made another mental note to get some better sweat-wicking pants.) During crescent lunge, I hooked my elbow outside my front leg for a twist, and I was sure I had wrung sweat out of my clothes onto my mat. Was everyone else sweating this much?

And the shaking. My arms shook during the long plank holds. During warriors, I thought my legs were tired, but my shoulders gave out first, exhausted from holding my arms up parallel to the floor.

By the time we got to backbends, I was wiped out. I wanted to lie on the floor and skip wheel, a pose I hadn't done since childhood. Pushing my hands and feet into the floor so my body made a rainbow shape was asking far more than I had left in me.

But somehow, I convinced myself to do it.

YOGA STYLES

As yoga has grown in popularity, varying styles of yoga have proliferated. Following is a outline of the basic styles, though the best way to understand them is to read the description and then talk to studio teachers. Be willing to try a few styles and studios before you decide on a practice that is right for you.

FLOW: Flow is a vigorous, physical practice. Ashtanga is the original style of flow, which includes elements where you practice moving one breath per pose. Any flow practice moves your body in the yoga poses in sync with your breath. Vinyasa flow is a common description for a flow practice, indicating the class will link moving through poses with an inhale or an exhale. Power vinyasa flow mixes in longer held poses with the flow. Some styles work with a set sequence or order of poses, such as Ashtanga and Baptiste Power Yoga, while others will sequence to change the order of poses every time you go.

HATHA: All yoga is a hatha practice, which refers to the physical yoga poses, but these days *hatha* generally indicates a non-flow practice. In a hatha or hot hatha class, you'll typically find classes offered in intense heat, with mirrors to help you focus your gaze, and a set series of 26 poses that stay the same regardless of teacher.

IYENGAR: Iyengar Yoga is another practice that switches between poses but does not include a vinyasa flow connecting breath and poses together. It works deeply and slowly into alignment. An Iyengar practice uses many props, such as blocks and straps, and it fine-tunes alignment with long holds.

KUNDALINI: A practice that combines meditation, poses, mantras, and breathing techniques, Kundalini also can include chanting. It's a slower-paced style that generally includes a lot of time spent on breathwork and meditation.

RESTORATIVE/YIN: A restorative or yin class is geared for people recovering from intense athletic days, folks with injuries or other physical challenges, or anyone who wants to move at a slower, modified pace. Restorative yoga, sometimes referred to as gentle yoga, may include flowing through some poses, linking poses with breath, or simply doing holds with props. In a yin practice, you hold a pose for a longer period of time for a deeper release in your fascia, or connective tissue.

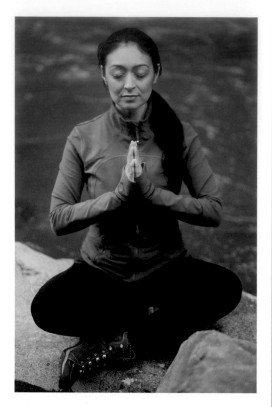

I was relieved when we stopped. Then the teacher started doing core work. Would this class never end? I couldn't touch my toes during the forward fold stretches and bemoaned my lack of flexibility. But once we reached final rest, when I could lie on the floor, my muscles soft, my mind stopped fixating on the sweat and my shaky muscles. I am pretty sure I took a short snooze. I am someone who is wired to be on the go, all the time. I tend to like intense, physically demanding classes. I didn't realize until final rest how much I needed to relax.

I knew right then that this was the style of yoga I wanted to do and the way I wanted to do it—work physically hard, sweat buckets, take a nap. It was dreamy.

The practice pressed the precise reset button I needed. I'd once worried I would get tired of yoga, that once I knew all the poses, it would bore me. I've taken thousands of yoga classes and am still fascinated by the practice, every time. Concentrating on sensations in your body, breathing, and staying focused makes anything you do physically inherently interesting.

The word *yoga* means union, a yoking of body and mind. It is an ancient, internal practice most widely known in the West for the physical practice of yoga poses. The spiritual and life-instructive elements of yoga can be found in ancient Indian teachings dating back 5,000 years. Research has suggested yoga has myriad benefits, including stress management, mental and emotional support, better sleep, and improved balance. Some studies have shown that it can relieve low-back pain and neck pain, too.

Yoga has grown enormously in popularity since my first power class, with styles ranging from seated meditation to a sweaty, music-filled vinyasa, and now includes yoga with goats or mixed with dance parties. I still love a power practice, but sometimes I prefer to rein in my energy and go to a more low-key class.

In that spirit, I went to a gentle yoga class designed for folks 50 and up.

Sitting on a bolster, a strap wrapped around my lower back and feet to help keep my pelvis and chest lifted upright, I noticed how focused my fellow students were. I could tell I would learn a few things from them. We were scattered throughout a community center gym, sitting on some combination of bolsters, blocks, and blankets. Nobody appeared distracted as yoga teacher Hiroko went around and checked on how everyone was set up on their bolster.

After our opening hip work, we moved into seated twists, again with many folks sitting on a block or a bolster to help tilt their pelvis forward for twists and forward folds. At first, I was distracted, reading a sign on the wall and not paying full attention to my twists. I reminded myself to follow the lead of my fellow students. I focused on my breath. We did a wide-legged forward fold, again rolling forward to tilt our pelvises forward, to make sure we were comfortable in the seat and to make sure we were taking advantage of the pose.

Afterward, we moved to our backs and lifted our legs into the air. I knew what was coming—core work. Hiroko had us lower one leg at a time, then lower both legs side to side for a twist and core challenge. The slow pace made the core engagement even more intense. When moving at Hiroko's pace, I couldn't use momentum to make it easier.

We turned over to our hands and knees to do our first downward-facing dog. Hiroko stopped us to explain how to rotate our shoulders and how to lengthen our spines in the pose. We did more core work on our hands and knees, extending legs and arms to challenge balance and

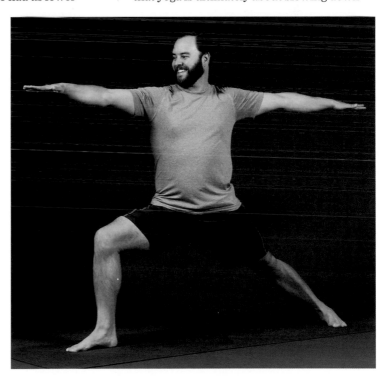

stability. By now, we were warm enough for backbends and moved down to the floor to add in some belly backbends.

The final push came in the last section of class, when we did warrior 2, triangle, and side angle. The intensity level increased here as we worked on leg strength and stability, and Hiroko checked on alignment to strengthen leg muscles and create joint stability. For balancing poses, Hiroko had us stand on one foot and open our shoulders for eagle pose. During seated shoulder openers, she told us to practice while watching television at home during an upcoming two-week class break.

Our final rest was quiet and sweet.

The class's slower pace reminded me that yoga is ultimately about slowing down mentally. We worked on both mobility and strength, and we focused our minds. While it was an all-levels gentle class, Hiroko said her regulars are strong, so she likes to challenge them, and I could tell. Taking the gentle yoga class with such a consistent, focused group of students was a lovely start to the day, both physically and mentally.

GET STARTED WITH YOGA

Take an intro class at a community center or yoga studio and go to class once a week for two weeks. See the "Yoga Styles" sidebar to determine what style of yoga might be the best fit for you.

BEFORE YOU GO

Equipment: Yoga mat, sweat towel, comfortable clothes to move in.
Cost: Drop-in fees at a community center or studio range from $8 to $25 per class. Check your local gym to see if classes are offered.

CHALLENGE YOURSELF

Try a few types of yoga (see sidebar) until you find a style that you like; then see if you can commit to that style of practice. Aim for these goals as your practice grows more advanced:

Level Up: Move up to all-levels classes and take two classes a week to start to understand the form and what it's like to learn from different teachers.
Reach Goal: Go to three or four classes a week. Observe the shift in your mental space when you practice more regularly and what you

can learn about poses by going to class more frequently.
Adventure Goal: Take a workshop that breaks down a particular pose or style. Much of your deeper learning will come with this kind of detailed instruction and plenty of practice.

QUICK TIPS

- Prepare to be physically challenged by poses as well as to stretch areas of your body that get tight and tense from sitting. If you're looking for a practice more focused on relaxation, take a slower style.
- Breathing is an essential component of a yoga practice. Even if you can't do a few poses, focus on breathing to help you relax and stay present.
- If you're going to a heated practice, bring a sweat towel plus an extra towel for your mat so you're not distracted by sliding around on your mat.
- Look to others in class for alignment help, and try not to get caught up in comparison. The goal is to feel your body in the poses and to notice what alignment keeps you healthy and safe. If you are injured, tell a teacher before class so they can support you with modifications. While teachers generally offer options to accommodate different experience levels in most classes, intro classes are still the best place to learn.

DISCOVERY: *Yoga*

	IST	2ND	3RD
DATE			
DURATION			
RATING (I TO 5 STARS)	★ ★ ★ ★ ★	★ ★ ★ ★ ★	★ ★ ★ ★ ★

How did you feel physically during your first yoga class? Did you embrace it? Or did you resist the poses or criticize how you did during a pose?

What did yoga feel like in your body the next day? Were you sore? Did you feel new muscles? Did anything shift in your relationship with your physical body? What did you learn from the challenge of the practice?

What kind of intention did you set at the start of class? What did you notice from setting an intention?

What did you notice about the conversations you have with yourself in yoga class?

Swing Dance

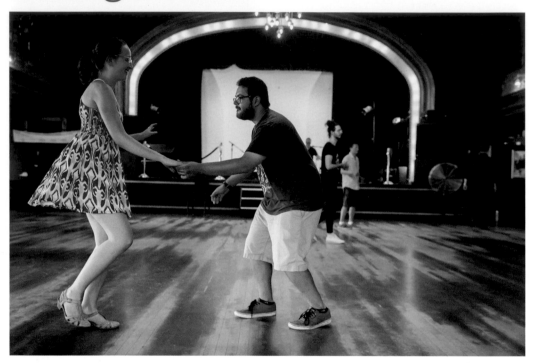

The best thing about swing is you can learn the basics in 30 minutes. Even less-than-coordinated dancers like me can pick up the steps fast and feel semicompetent to join an open swing dance session. On the flip side, it takes far more practice than a 30-minute class to master swing—when I figured this out, I watched my dreams of sweet swing stardom go *poof*.

I took a class in East Coast swing, considered the most accessible type of swing.

East Coast is so accommodating that the dance studio I chose teaches 30-minute intro classes right before its regular open swing dances, held several times a week for people eager for swing time with live music.

Dance, and in particular social dance, can make a big difference in how you live out your final years. A 2003 study on mental acuity published in *The New England Journal of Medicine* showed that out of 11 physical activities, only social dancing was associated

OR TRY . . . SALSA

Of all the things I thought I might appreciate about salsa dancing—and I liked so many elements—holding hands with a stranger was not one of them. But the "social" aspect of social dance is actually one of the sweetest parts of taking salsa.

In salsa class, after warm-ups and before partnering up, we built on the basic salsa step, which, for the follower, is a step back with the right foot, back to center, then a step forward with the left foot and back to center. We danced to music and added a spin. Once I figured out the mechanics of a spin, it felt simple.

When we followers paired up with the leads to practice, it got more complex. Leads rotated their partners, with only a few steps per person. Many of my leads had furrowed brows, their lips silently counting numbers in sync with the music as they led me through the basic step and tossed in spins.

Next, we added in a walk past our partners, then turned around. The step was simple, so our teachers showed us "styling," with fun arm movements to add flair. As usual, when I did it alone, it was simple. Throw in a partner, and things could go in any direction.

Our instructors then added the cumbia—a basic step that goes side to side—and new arm positions, encouraging followers to make good arm contact with our leads so they could move us more easily.

Weaving in new steps and arms ramped up the challenge, but my feet knew what to do. I began to see more leads smiling, even as some still whisper-counted to themselves.

I longed for the hip- and arm-flashing styling of our teachers. That will take practice, which I can't wait to do.

with a reduced risk of developing dementia for people 75 years old and up.

At our class, a surprisingly large group of students gathered around our swing instructor, Mark. Some were dressed in ties and hats or retro dresses; I suspected they had been to swing before, and I was mildly jealous they looked so good. Note to self: Wear a cool retro dress next time.

First, Mark showed us the basic step: rock, step, step. Rock back on the right foot (for followers), then forward on the left, step the right foot out and step back on the left. Simple. He had us grab partners in a giant circle, and we practiced the step, rotating through new partners quickly.

One of my partners, whom I suspected had done swing before, got a little fancy, spinning me out, then back in. I can't say it was a success; I was confused about my feet, and they got tangled. I was on the wrong foot by the time I got back to my partner. Womp-womp. But my partner was on target; next, we learned how to do swing-outs.

Once Mark showed us how to move our feet, I disentangled my footwork and had fun again. I practiced with various partners, spinning out under their arm, then back in. I grew more confident about my ability to get back to my partner without issues.

Mark also showed us how to turn in to our partners, another slick move, which was more challenging but added pizzazz to our core moves.

Our final technique for the evening was the freeze, where each person stomped down on their front foot and froze in place. Just make sure you stomp away from your partner, he reminded us. I loved the freeze—the stylized move made me feel like a legit swing dancer.

After 30 minutes practicing with our safe, nonthreatening intro class, Mark unleashed

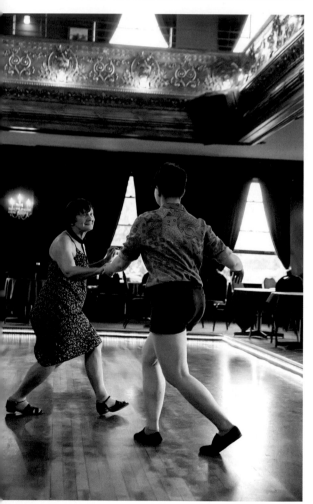

us into the social dance. I realized I had three moves and the other dancers had a whole lot more.

Three is better than one, but once the real dancers moved onto the floor, I felt shy. I danced with a couple of intro students and then met some people who knew how to string several moves together. I got a taste of Lindy Hop with one partner, who swung me around fast. I learned the Chicago slide from another and watched him groove comfortably to the big band music. Sometimes I stood on the sidelines watching experienced dancers twirl each other around. I also contemplated whether I should take a real class that would teach me more moves.

It was as if Mark had read my mind. Not long after, he reached out to say he wanted to teach me to Lindy Hop, and to show me it's not hard. He said he could teach me the dance in one hour, and he used phrases like "the most joyful dance of all time" and "no previous dance experience."

Dance. On.

Lindy Hop evolved in the 1920s and '30s and is considered the original swing dance. Most quintessential swing moves you see are variations of Lindy Hop, which is well loved in the partner dance world. Athletes, and especially runners, like it because it is athletic, with a lot of hopping around, and it doesn't require a lot of technique to master the basic moves, though once you get into jumps, I can't vouch that it's easy.

After an hour of hopping around, I can attest to both the ease of learning the early moves and the constant, energetic movement that is an essential part of Lindy Hop. You don't need any previous dance background, as Mark said. If you can run and you can hop, you can Lindy Hop. Time to toss all those excuses out the door.

When I met Mark for a class, he zoomed through the essentials. We started off with basic rhythms, clapping first, stomping our feet, then moving our feet to the rhythm. The triple steps required for the Lindy Hop step tested my sense of rhythm at first, as I struggled to coordinate my feet to the tempo, but I wasn't lost, or at least that's what I told myself.

Swing dance becomes even more joyful when working with a skilled partner, and I was dancing with an experienced teacher, which meant I could handle a swing-out with little warning.

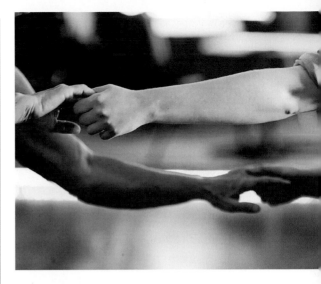

Lindy Hop has three gears, Mark explained, and once you learn them, you can keep up with any partner or any song. When Mark stayed in one gear, I could keep up as he threw out occasional new moves, but when he switched between two steps and mixed up the rhythm, I got confused and ended up on the wrong foot on the wrong beat. But Mark took it all in stride, reminding me to look at him and follow his lead.

Finally, I learned the Charleston, which adds kicks on each foot to the basic Lindy Hop step. Though it was technically harder, I felt jazzy doing the kick. We hopped from foot to foot with little kicks forward and back. I wished I had worn a sequined, black-fringed dress, a matching headband, and elegant elbow-length gloves.

When I asked how I would know mid-dance when it was time to switch into the Charleston, Mark said it's obvious—he would move from a smooth step to hopping up and down. I did my best, and when he suddenly went from moving me around the floor to bopping up and down, I jumped around. During the

Charleston, he tossed in a swing with double kicks, and suddenly I wanted to bop around all night long, dancing my heart out.

Most partner dances use a traditional leader-and-follower format, but Lindy Hop is more open to personal expression. Either partner can throw in their own stylistic moves at any moment during the dance. Still, a great lead will make all the difference when learning to Lindy Hop.

For our final dance, Mark told me I could either do what he did or keep doing what I had learned. My brain was in a hopping tizzy, and I decided to stick with what I'd learned until it was secured in muscle memory.

We started off with the familiar step-step-triple step. Just when I had gotten my groove, Mark added big hip swings and some jazzy steps to the basic moves. I couldn't help but join in and attempt to get a little sass in my hips and wave my hands around. Other times, Mark's steps were more complicated, and I stayed with my reliable triple steps while he added in some pizzazz.

In case you missed the message, Lindy Hopping is joy embodied. Once you know the Lindy Hop gears, Mark said, work on your moves at the weekly swing dances. Sounds like a worthy, and fun, challenge.

GET STARTED SWING DANCING

Look for class offerings at local dance studios or community centers. Take a single intro class to learn basic swing. You may find a one-off class where you can check out the dance and see if you like it.

QUICK TIPS

- Swing dance is more fun when you dress up, so consider wearing a swingy skirt, heels, or a dapper tie for an open social dance.
- Don't worry if you don't come with a partner; you'll rotate through leads and follows in class.
- If you can, go to a dance and see if you can learn from a more experienced dancer, practice your basics, and experiment with new moves.

BEFORE YOU GO

Equipment: Comfortable clothes and shoes to dance in.
Cost: Varies, depending on if you go to a community center or a dance studio, or if you are taking an introductory series. Fees typically range from $5 to $15 per class.

CHALLENGE YOURSELF

It takes some time to get used to dancing with others, but if you commit to doing it regularly, you may find that it's the most joyful part of social dance. If you love your first class, try these:

Level Up: Commit to a full class series, which often goes for a month or up to eight classes. You'll get so much more out of doing the dance regularly and practicing every week.
Reach Goal: Go to an open swing session if there is one near you. Test out your skills on an evening out.
Adventure Goal: Take an advanced swing class, and learn to string together more moves at a time and even do aerial moves, where your feet come off the floor and you learn what it feels like to fly—or to fly others—while dancing.

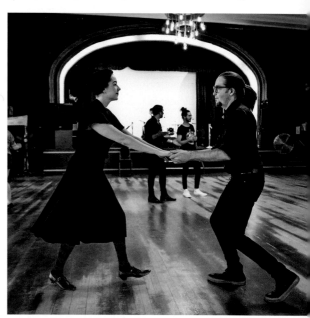

DISCOVERY: *Swing Dance*

	1ST	2ND	3RD
DATE			
DURATION			
RATING (1 TO 5 STARS)	★ ★ ★ ★ ★	★ ★ ★ ★ ★	★ ★ ★ ★ ★

How did you feel the first time you started learning the basic steps for swing? Did you feel clumsy or like you were off the beat, or did you have more fun than you thought?

Muscle memory is a glorious thing. How did you feel the second time you went swing dancing?

What did you learn or observe about dancing with a partner? Were you nervous to hold a stranger's hand? What did you learn about human touch?

What surprised you most about swing dancing, from the actual steps to partner dancing to how you felt afterward?

Month **6**

Ultimate

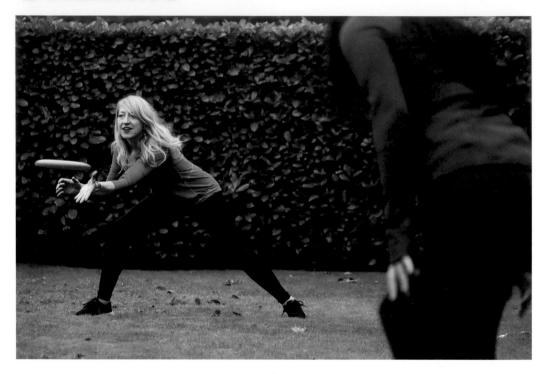

We gathered around, a motley crew of eight. Olivia, our ultimate expert, was the only one with any experience with the sport—as a member of a team that placed sixth at nationals, no less.

I'd recruited Olivia to help me learn to play ultimate. Team sports and I are not friends, nor even on somewhat friendly terms. They are uncharted territory to me, due to a childhood spent on the ice and tennis courts, neither of which count in my mind as team sports. By the time I reached the adult world, I wasn't interested in hustling around a sports field with a team, trying to communicate well with teammates, thinking strategy on a field, and running like a fiend.

But if I was going to throw myself into team-building, high-fiving territory, ultimate seemed like the easiest way to go, as far as technical skills were concerned—more so than basketball, volleyball, or soccer. And ultimate is a no-contact team sport, which I prefer. When playing, teams pass an ultimate Frisbee disc between them to score against the opposing team.

In addition to providing a major cardiovascular challenge with constant sprinting and maneuvering around the opposing team, the benefits of ultimate, as with all team sports, extend into the social and psychological realm. Studies show that being on a team can improve your overall health; one study by the *Journal of the American Medical Association Pediatrics* showed that doing team sports in grades 7 to 12 led to better mental health as adults, with a lower likelihood of depression, especially in males, in addition to building endurance and increasing bone density and muscle strength overall.

Olivia originally gave me the option to play pickup ultimate at a large local park where people play with other interested folks, but playing a team sport with strangers sounded like a childhood nightmare come to life. Now that I'm an adult, I chose to opt out. Instead, she agreed to help me round up a few friends for a casual pickup game on our own, which sounded less scary and even potentially fun.

I had a sneaking suspicion some of our group, an athletic crew, would pick up ultimate quickly. I had more than a passing suspicion that I would not be one of them. But I like to think I have hustle and determination, so I hoped that would be good enough.

Olivia gave us the rundown for a game of mini-ultimate, or three players on three, as opposed to the standard seven per team for a regular ultimate game. We had eight people, so we made four on four work, splitting up into coed teams.

Olivia put down bright-orange cones to mark off the goals and gave us a primer in some ultimate rules. We huddled to discuss which team was headed to which goal, separated to discuss who was guarding whom, and then we were off.

Ultimate is a fast game, from the speed of the disc to the constant action on the field. I could barely keep up at first, both with the new-to-me rules and especially with defense. I struggled to focus on what was happening with the disc at any given time. You can't run once you catch the disc—you have to find an open teammate to throw it to—and you also have a limit of five seconds to do something with the disc. The guard counts down on the person holding the disc, who has to throw; otherwise they get penalized. When guarding, I kept forgetting to do the five count; I also tried to run at least once while holding the disc.

Guarding is difficult in general, but it is especially tough when keeping an eye on a spitfire like my friend Natalie, whom I'd recruited to play. I knew she was athletic. During ultimate, I felt like I was chasing a whirling dervish around the field as she darted this way and that to get open to catch the disc. She, in turn, kept waving her arms at me when guarding me, and I could barely see around her to find an open teammate to throw to. Relentless was an understatement.

Then there's the technical side of throwing and catching—not my strength—and the fact that turnovers happen fast in ultimate; drop the disc and the opposing team takes possession of it. Which led me to my first impression of ultimate, and team sports in general: vigorous, with a dose of insanity. Like running at full sprint almost the entire time. Since I avoid running, this was intense.

The question that kept crossing my mind was: Are all team sports this hard? Quick answer: yes.

I soon realized I'm better at catching than throwing, especially when the disc is thrown directly to me. To advance down the field, it helps to understand the dynamics of team strategy and throwing the disc to the spot you expect a teammate to be, rather than where they started. I understood that kind of throw in theory. I failed to chase and catch a few throws sent down the field by others who understand how to put the strategy into play. Seeing where the disc was going and putting myself in the correct position was a skill under development.

We also mixed up the team members. This switch kept things balanced, but it also created confusion—or was that only for me? I could never remember who was on my team or figure out where I should be. I almost shouted in triumph a couple of times when a former teammate intercepted a pass.

Most of us had never played ultimate, and it showed at the beginning. Throughout the game, people's skills improved. Interceptions happened on purpose! People threw with more accuracy! We learned to throw low, rather than high, decreasing the likelihood of an interception. In the heat of the moment, I often forgot there were two ways to throw the disc—the traditional way I'd played Frisbee growing up (throwing it from my chest) or chucking it (holding the disk with my palm up and flicking my wrist). I had a long list of skills to work on.

You might assume that I hated ultimate, that every moment of the game was torture. I was shocked when I realized mid-game I was loving it. I couldn't imagine a better way to spend an evening than running around on a field with a bunch of my friends. Perhaps I wouldn't like it as much if I had to play with strangers or if there was more on the line, like a national championship, but when I played with friends who were a combination of friendly and fiercely competitive, we had a blast. We guarded, ran at top speed, laughed, and had a ball.

I had so much fun that the hour flew by; I was a sweaty, panting mess by the end.

I concluded that team sports and I could potentially like each other, or at least have a mini-crush, though it will take a few more games to seal the friendship.

GET STARTED WITH ULTIMATE

Practice your skills with a friend once or twice a week. Get a disc, get in some throws and catches, and get comfortable running.

QUICK TIPS

- Find someone who can show you the basics, either in an intro class or at a beginner pickup game where you can learn the ropes.
- As you would for any team sport, practice some of the skills required and make sure you understand the basic rules for ultimate before jumping onto the field.
- Be prepared for occasional eruptions of competitiveness on the field!

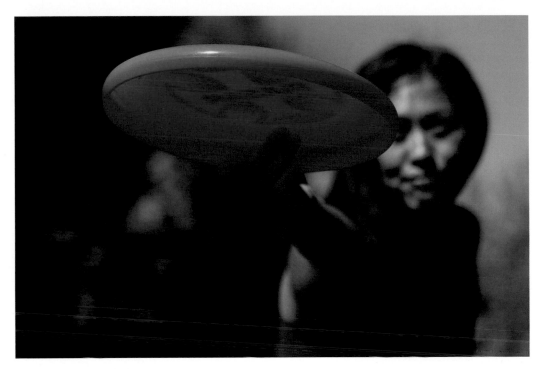

BEFORE YOU GO

Equipment: An ultimate disc (different from a regular Frisbee), clothes suitable for running and sweating, sneakers or cleats.

Cost: Free if playing pickup; costs start around $30 to join a recreation league.

CHALLENGE YOURSELF

Once you've dialed in your skills throwing and catching, add in more people for another layer of fun and challenge. Try these ideas:

Level Up: Gather some friends for a pickup game and learn some of the rules and skills in a friendly, hopefully noncompetitive environment. Do this at least once.

Reach Goal: Look for a beginner pickup game or a beginner league, and dive into the challenge of advancing your skills and playing a game with strangers.

Adventure Goal: Join a league to have a regular team, and play one to two times a week.

DISCOVERY: *Ultimate*

	1ST	2ND	3RD
DATE			
DURATION			
RATING (1 TO 5 STARS)	★ ★ ★ ★ ★	★ ★ ★ ★ ★	★ ★ ★ ★ ★

Is the idea of a team sport intimidating? What comes up for you at the thought of learning to play ultimate or another team sport?

If ultimate was new to you, what did you discover about trying something you have no experience with?

How did you feel after your first game, pickup or otherwise? Did you feel physically challenged? What did you learn about strategy when playing with a group of people on a team?

After a game, how did you feel about playing with other people? If you missed a catch or a throw was off, what did you observe about your own reaction?

RECOVERY: *Healing from Injury*

The pain started in the middle of the night. The spasms in my mid-back were so excruciating that the pain woke me up. I couldn't get back to sleep.

The next day, walking made the pain worse. It was so intense, I was nauseous. The pain moved from my mid-back and shot up and under my ribs. I gave up on my day and laid on the couch. But resting didn't make me feel better. The pain was so agonizing, I knew I needed help.

I had felt twinges in my back earlier in the week during back squats. After I'd used a roller on the knots, the spasms disappeared. I assumed my body had taken care of the problem. When I lifted again a few days later, I felt another round of spasms. I woke up in the middle of the night with the worst injury I had experienced in years.

Since my last injury four years prior, my approach to healing had transformed. I'd learned the most important thing to do is to seek help so the injury becomes a temporary hurdle rather than a mountain you have to keep climbing the rest of your days. If you're proactive, you can leave the injury behind rather than live with it.

That previous injury had happened when I was trying to stay on a wall at a rock climbing gym. My hip made a little pop as I lifted my foot and placed it on the climbing hold, but I ignored it. I put all my weight onto my foot, and the shooting pain in my groin shocked me.

I made it to the top and climbed a couple more routes, but the pain would not go away. That night, it worsened. In the morning, it was excruciating. I spent the day icing and moping. I figured the healing protocol known as RICE (rest, ice, compress, elevate) would take care of it. I didn't know studies show movement, not rest, aids recovery from injury.

I took a full week off before doing an upper body workout. Two weeks later, I did yoga, being careful not to aggravate my groin. Three weeks post-injury, things were almost back to normal, although I backed off whenever there was a twinge. I used my foam roller daily.

I did not see a professional.

I thought my body bounced back.

I now know the truth. Recovery needs expert help. Instead of fully healing, my body accommodated the injury and created new movement patterns to protect the injured muscles. Since I never had a professional retrain those muscles to fire the way they're intended right after the injury, I now live with hip flare-ups, a twisted mid-back, and glutes that are sluggish on one side. It's been a long, uncomfortable lesson that still requires monthly chiropractic visits.

My new approach—when injured, call professionals. ASAP.

After my first sleepless night with my injured back, I went to Sam Hammer, an orthopedic massage therapist, who had one opening that day. I hobbled into his office. He examined how I moved and prodded my back. I had twisted a couple of vertebrae in my mid-back, he said. The body doesn't like it when your spine is out of alignment. Tell me about it.

Sam worked on the muscle spasms in my obliques and around my ribs. I winced from the intensity. I asked what would happen if I didn't deal with the pain now, and he said this sort of injury can lead to herniated discs. Eyes wide, I made a follow-up appointment.

That night, my back still seized. My lifting coach recommended heat and rolling my back on tennis balls to get blood into the injured area. I clutched my heating pad to me like a security blankie, unwilling to go anywhere without its soothing warmth. I rolled my back in the middle of the night when I couldn't sleep. I took mild painkillers for temporary relief.

As the days dragged on, I wondered if I would ever feel strong again. I had renewed compassion for people suffering from debilitating injuries. I brooded over whether this was the end of my movement career.

I went to a float tank, buoyed by saltwater, which relieved the tension in my back. I basked in the heat lamp at acupuncture, with needles in my back and my legs. I went back to Hammer, who noted that an old head injury from college that impacted my vision may have affected how I hold my neck, then torqued my rib cage and created stiffness and weakness in my mid-back.

Despite all the time and money I spent, I wasn't sure if these treatments would help me heal. I could barely cook dinner, let alone work. But seven days in, a miracle happened—I slept through the night. In the morning, the pain had lessened. A day later, it was almost gone. I wanted to jump for joy, except I didn't want to injure myself again.

I went back to yoga, modifying my practice. I added light weightlifting into my routine. My chiropractor adjusted my spine, ribs, and neck and worked on my squat technique.

I could breathe again.

It's been several years since that injury. My back hasn't spoken up since then. I built back up to heavy weightlifting. My hip, however, nags me, a reminder of what happens when I don't take care of an injury.

I can't say I was happy to be injured, but I'm grateful for what I learned—about healing from injury and about my body—and ecstatic to sleep through the night again.

Month 7

Kickboxing

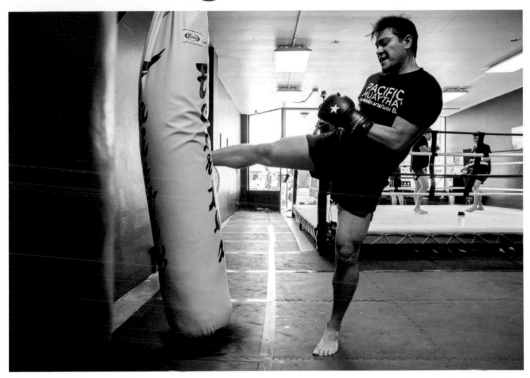

I expected kickboxing to be hard. I'm into a gasping-for-air, limbs-shaking kind of challenge. Twenty-four minutes into an hour-long class, breathing heavily and dripping sweat, I looked at the clock and decided challenge was overrated.

When I'd looked around for a kickboxing class, I wanted the real deal. I found a martial arts studio that offered fitness kickboxing for building strength. When I called to ask about the class, I was told the main difference between the fitness class and real kickboxing was I wouldn't get hit in the face.

Growing up with a sister and skipping the rough-and-tumble route of team sports, I've never lived in a world where I was pushed, let alone punched or kicked. I felt good about the no-face-punching rule but wondered if it was an indicator that the physical intensity would be high. I decided to try it anyway.

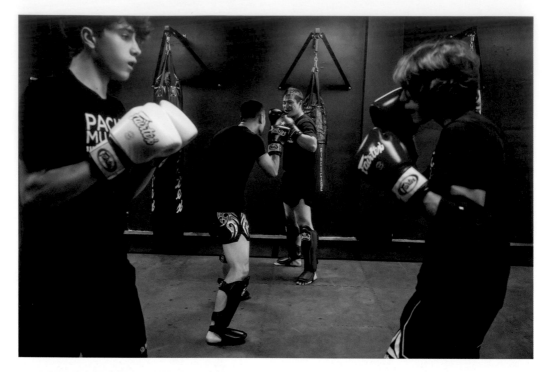

The studio was clean and bright, with punching bags and plenty of room. Once I got set up with some red kickboxing gloves, I was ready for class, at least on the outside. Our teacher, Silas, started us out with a fast warm-up, including jumping jacks, squats, and push-ups. After a brief stretch, he rolled out freestanding black punching bags. It was time to take our aggression out on the bags.

We started with basic punching combos, working the jab, cross, and hook. I took cues from other students, who punched their bags with fierce cries and grunts. Silas threw in additional moves, including half burpees in between punches for our combos, then let us go at it for a few minutes at a time.

My heart rate went up fast during the combos, but I was focused on getting all my angst and aggression out on the bag. Silas walked around giving tips, showing me how to pivot on my standing foot for side kicks. He advised me to use my shin instead of the top of my foot as added protection from the repeated kicks.

Then the combos got longer. Despite water breaks, I realized the difficulty of the class was rising. We added hooks and ducks to our combos. We did more burpees. My shoulders started to ache. After we added front kicks for speed and changed our burpees to core work on the floor, my shoulders ached so much I was grateful to stop punching for a few counts, even if it was to do core.

Just when I thought I couldn't punch my bag any more, Silas added in blitzes, where we punched and kicked our bags as hard as possible for 30 seconds at a time, with 10-second breaks. The people around me pummeled their bags. With a sigh, I told myself I was tough, and I went at it. About 15 minutes before the end of class, I got my hopes up that the punching and kicking torture was almost over.

Silas announced it was time to punch our bags 100 times, kick them another 50, and then do 10 push-ups. I stared back at him. It wasn't over. Not even close.

I dug in deep and did all the reps in the sequence, twice. Right as I was about to keel over on the floor, time was up. We did partner work to close the class, with jabs and crosses, before "cooling down" with push-ups.

The truth is, I secretly adore a punishing class. Kickboxing class ranked high on punishment, resulting in shaky legs, exhausted shoulders, and core muscles that hurt the next day. You'd think I would have been satisfied after that first kickboxing class. Nope. I wanted to test the waters with the next level of class—training like competitive kickboxers do. But if I'd been told in advance that I'd actually be training with competitive kickboxers, I might not have shown up.

Everyone appeared to be sweating already when I arrived at a local competitive Muay Thai gym for class. Had they already worked out, and was the foundations class I was about to take a cooldown?

I soon learned they not only came early to work out but also stayed after for more sparring. Who are these people? My only explanation for them—not normal.

I had chosen a gym that teaches Muay Thai, or Thai boxing. Kickboxing uses just punches and kicks, while Muay Thai, which falls under the umbrella of kickboxing, adds in strikes using knees and elbows.

Boxing conditioning will whip you into shape, fast. Be prepared to move the entire class. Kickboxing improves fitness, power, flexibility, and agility, according to one study of men in their twenties who trained three days a week for five weeks. Plus, it's similar to high-intensity interval training (HIIT), with short stretches of intense, repetitive moves like punching the bag or sparring with a partner. Some research shows that brief stretches of HIIT can offer similar gains in heart and lung health as longer stretches of less-intense exercise.

I can also attest that punching or kicking bags (or consenting opponents, usually holding mitts) is an excellent way to release stress.

Coach Kim Nguyen started us jumping rope. About two minutes in, my calves were burning while everyone else was skipping leisurely, adding tricks, jumping one foot at a time, and playing around. I figured out I had to take breaks on my own because they don't give many.

Our warm-ups were so vigorous—with fast sprints back and forth over mats, burpees, bear crawls, high knees, and jumping in place—that I worried about the workout. I know boxing requires bursts of speed and power, but did we need to put this much effort in this early?

After working on splits to stretch hips (boxers do splits?), we moved to shadowboxing, working on punches, jabs, and hooks. I learned the form for using my knee, thrusting my knee forward, and also how to do a controlled kick.

Coach Kim stopped at each person, watching their form. He corrected me on how to spin my hips and how to keep one hand up by my face for protection, before saying, "Nice work, Nicole," and moving on. I was happy to take any encouragement as the competitive boxers around me danced and whipped feet and gloves in the direction of imaginary opponents.

For sparring, Coach Kim partnered me with Florence, the other only woman in class that day. I was relieved to work with a woman, though I soon learned Florence had plenty of bite in her kick. First, she had me wear her gloves while she held mitts to defend against me doing different combinations, including jab, punch, hook, and jab, punch, hook, elbow. The regular boxing combinations felt familiar from previous boxing classes. Florence reminded me to keep my hips facing forward and to protect my face with my glove. The elbow was the hardest move, as I tried to slide my feet forward and

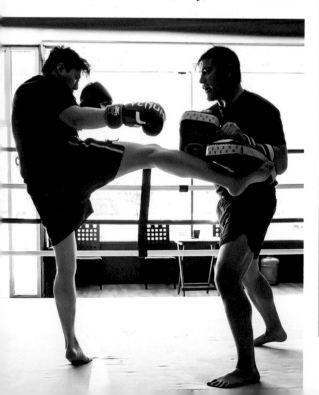

throw my weight into my elbow and into Florence's mitt.

Learning to knee an opponent was tough. It felt awkward pushing my hips forward and kneeing into the mitts. The kick was easier, with a sharp turn and whip of one leg into the pads.

After practicing set combinations, we went into free sparring, where Florence instructed me on the order of kicks and punches. She threw new combinations at me and surprised me when she told me to kick and knee with my left leg.

Um, I only know how to do that move with my right leg.

Florence encouraged me to keep at it until I ended with 10 kicks on each leg. I was seriously beat.

But now it was my turn to hold the mitts, which seemed like an easy task. It was not. This was a new skill, punching back when Florence pummeled the mitts and making sure I held the mitts in the right place so neither of us got hurt. Florence kicked and kneed with massive force. Halfway through, my shoulders were so tired, I could barely hold the mitts up and defend against her.

Just when I thought we were done, Coach Kim told us to put down our mitts and gloves and come back to the mats for a final round of planks, mountain runners, high knees, and burpees. I was ready to collapse. I looked around, and the other boxers at least looked human now, with tired eyes and sweat pouring down their faces.

The atmosphere at the studio was focused, without a lot of joking around, and by the end, we'd all bonded over the intensity of the class. You can go to a gym to kickbox for fitness, or you can learn competitive Thai boxing. Either way, you'll work out stress and aggression, build up your endurance, and be humbled.

GET STARTED KICKBOXING

Find a local kickboxing class and go once a week. See how you feel punching, kicking, and getting your heart rate up.

QUICK TIPS

- If you're interested in just conditioning and shadowboxing, look for a kickboxing class and be prepared to get your heart pumping.
- If you're interested in sparring, whether against a partner or potentially to compete, consider looking for a Muay Thai studio to get the full competitive experience.
- Some martial arts studios require uniforms for classes. Call ahead to find out.

BEFORE YOU GO

Equipment: Boxing gloves, comfortable shoes, clothes to move in (or a uniform, if you're at a martial arts studio that requires one). Studios have the equipment for sale.
Cost: Depends on the studio; drop-in classes range from $10 to $20.

CHALLENGE YOURSELF

Be prepared to move, whether you're joining a basics class or heading to a more advanced level. After a couple weekly sessions, kick it up with these goals:

Level Up: Go to a kickboxing class twice a week, and see how you feel.
Reach Goal: If there's an intermediate class, consider moving up to a higher level of kickboxing. Otherwise, start to increase your endurance in class by taking fewer breaks.
Adventure Goal: Look for a competitive kickboxing or Muay Thai gym and see how you feel in a foundations class.

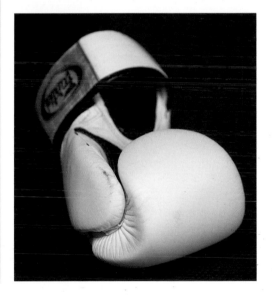

DISCOVERY: *Kickboxing*

	1ST	2ND	3RD
DATE			
DURATION			
RATING (1 TO 5 STARS)	★ ★ ★ ★ ★	★ ★ ★ ★ ★	★ ★ ★ ★ ★

If, like me, you didn't grow up roughhousing, what did you discover about kicking or punching a bag or a human? Did you like kicking and punching another person? How did you feel about someone kicking or punching you?

What did you find out about your endurance—or potentially the need to develop it—from an hour-long kickboxing class?

Did anything about the class surprise you? What was it?

Month 7

Trail Running

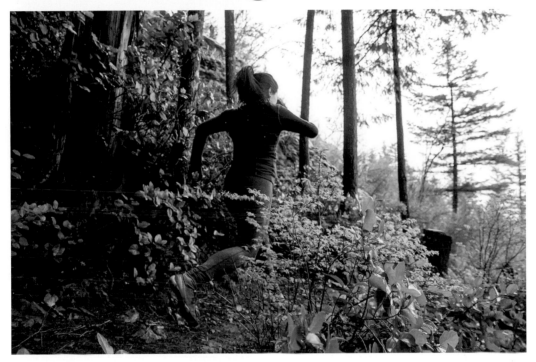

Running is a sport that ranks among my least favorite ways to sweat. My running block has been so big and lasted for so long, I thought maybe it had more to do with running on flat surfaces like streets. Perhaps I need to run in the woods, I told myself. It can't be worse than running on a sidewalk, right?

Soon, I found myself jumping over roots and dashing around sharp rocks, with my running coach telling me to keep my eyes ahead 15 feet. If you look up while trail running, you can see obstacles and flow through them, Malcolm said as he ran easily through the woods with me. I nodded as I huffed behind him and tried to flow through the trails without falling over.

I went to Malcolm to get tips on trail running technique. He's a longtime runner, including road running, and teaches various running courses, including a trail running class with some circuit training to build strength.

OR TRY . . . TRAINING FOR A 5K

I ran a 5K, once. I was the running leg of a triathlon.

I did it partly to try to get over a serious mental block about running. I ran twice a week for four weeks beforehand and called it "training." It wasn't the worst experience I've ever had—I also have not run a race since.

Running coach Beth Baker works with people like me who are active and fit and can't stand running. Some resistance is based in human biology, she said. Your brain goes into fight-or-flight mode on a run, thinking you're in danger. New runners, especially fit ones, run too fast, refuse to walk, and get tired. You have to build endurance.

You can train for a 5K in roughly a month, Beth said. Go for a walk/run for 30 to 40 minutes three to four times a week. Use small visual goals, like street signs, to motivate yourself in small chunks. Go slow, and walk if you need to.

One way to get over fight or flight is to run in a pack. But group running can bring up another worry—nobody wants to be last.

Beth understands. "In a primal sense, if you're dead last, you're picked off," she said. "Get a buddy so no one ends last. Buddies also help with pacing. If you can't talk, you're running too fast."

If you decide to train for a 5K, your first goal is to finish the race. After that, your goals may change to running the entire time, going faster, or running a half marathon.

For long runs, "the first three miles are the hardest," Beth said. "Once people get past that, they can run forever; it's just training your body."

I'll stick with the 5K, thanks.

Runners face obstacles whether they run in the forest or on city streets, where challenges include cracks in sidewalks, cars whizzing past on busy streets, or having to calculate traffic lights. If there's no sidewalk, runners need to stay visible and be able to spot cars by running against traffic.

A 2014 study in the *Journal of American College of Cardiology* of a group of more than 55,000 men and women ages 18 to 100 found that over the course of 15 years, those who ran 5 to 10 minutes a day at a moderate or even low-intensity pace were less likely to die from cardiovascular disease compared to those who didn't run at all.

For many folks, running is an alluring combination of physical intensity mixed with time outside in fresh air, the meditative element of a longer run, and a runner's high—the irresistible release of endorphins that comes from consistent training on longer runs.

But it takes time to build up endurance and strength, regardless of whether you run in the streets or in the woods. When starting out, it helps to run based on time rather than distance, though you can still track how far you went. As your endurance builds, you can look into basing your runs on mileage and speed.

Malcolm started me on an easy run through a local park rich with trees and trails, where he extolled the virtues of trail running, with its softer surface that is easier on the feet and joints.

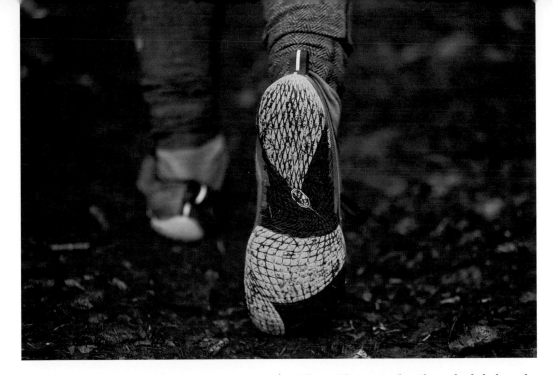

Trail runners have to adapt more to handle conditions, he said, starting with the constant shift between up- and downhill. On the uphill, he showed me how to lift my fists slightly higher than my elbows and pump my arms faster to move my legs faster. Sometimes, it is more efficient to power walk uphill than run, he said, taking big strides that use different leg muscles than running. During one particularly long, steady uphill, I was relieved to drop back to a power walk.

On the downhill, he told me to loosen my arms and let my fists drop a little below my elbows to open up my stride. You can lean back to brake on the way down, but leaning forward at the ankle takes advantage of gravity to churn down the hills; it requires strength and agility.

Learning to flow while running on a trail—that is, moving with obstacles instead of letting them affect your pace—was more technical. You move your legs and torso side to side on a trail, and you duck, bob, and weave, Malcolm said as he dodged a branch. When we approached a low fence that was partially down, he showed me how, if I looked far enough ahead, I could hurdle the fence. I argued that if you looked ahead, you could run around the fence instead of hurdling it and not slow down, too. He smiled and concurred it was an option.

Moving side to side requires lateral stability in your body. Malcolm showed me some balancing exercises to strengthen ankles and knees, such as standing with one foot directly in front of the other. Some people have trouble with even that; he encourages them to work on the exercise at home. Other movements included stepping back into a low lunge, then stepping the same leg forward into a lunge without stopping, which builds stability and strength in the hips.

For an added balance and strength challenge, Malcolm had me lift one leg to the side and back until my butt muscles engaged, and then slowly lower the standing leg into a squat. It's not easy to do without toppling over. You also can practice lateral shuffles, going side to side. Or stand on one leg and swing the other leg side to side, holding on to a tree if needed to balance. The lateral balancing work got me out of the tougher cross-training Malcolm does in class, such as push-ups on slopes, facing both up- and downhill, to build strength.

On the way back, we had a long downhill stretch. Malcolm wanted me to lean slightly forward. I liked the speed and felt like it was still relatively low impact, though my instincts went against angling my body forward on a downhill slope. Holding back and braking with my legs seemed safer, although it also seemed like it would be a more painful choice.

The trail run felt different from previous runs. Thinking of the run as an obstacle course kept my mind engaged on what was to come rather than on how much time I had left or how far I had to go, two thoughts that often get in my way when I run on sidewalks or a track. I also preferred the soft surface and the lower impact on my feet and joints.

Over the years, I've learned that whatever I don't want to do is the pathway to reach new levels of awareness and strength. Are you about to add running to break out of your usual regimen or to move more? Let's do it together.

GET STARTED TRAIL RUNNING

Head to a nearby park or trailhead and go for a 15-minute run once a week, just to see how it feels. Don't worry about distance; set a timer and go. Let yourself walk if you need to.

QUICK TIPS

- Get fitted for trail running shoes. When you get serious about trail running, it helps to find a shoe that you can wear consistently and has tread suitable for trails, especially if you plan to put in a lot of miles.
- Be safe when you run. If you run with headphones on, keep the volume turned to a level where you can still hear what's going on around you.

BEFORE YOU GO

Equipment: Trail running shoes, comfortable clothes, a supportive bra for women.
Cost: Free at local parks, although you may need to pay $5 to $10 for parking or day passes if you go to a state park.

CHALLENGE YOURSELF

Once you've motivated yourself to do a 15-minute run weekly, start to build your endurance for these milestones:

Level Up: Increase your run time to 30 minutes and go twice a week. Again, allow yourself to walk if you need to.
Reach Goal: Go three times a week for 30 minutes per run. Change your route to challenge your body with different terrain and scenery. If you're traveling, consider running while you're somewhere new.
Adventure Goal: Train to run a set distance, like a 10K. If there are trail races in your area, consider signing up for one.

DISCOVERY: *Trail Running*

	1ST	2ND	3RD
DATE			
DURATION			
RATING (1 TO 5 STARS)	★ ★ ★ ★ ★	★ ★ ★ ★ ★	★ ★ ★ ★ ★

What did you discover about trail running after you started to go once or twice a week?

What did you notice when you gave yourself permission to walk if you needed to?

What did you learn about the trail or park systems near your home after you started running? Running also travels well—what did you observe about places you visited by looking for trails and running?

After trail running regularly for a couple weeks, what have you noticed that has changed physically? What has shifted mentally? What did you notice about consistent time outside or in the woods?

Indoor Climbing

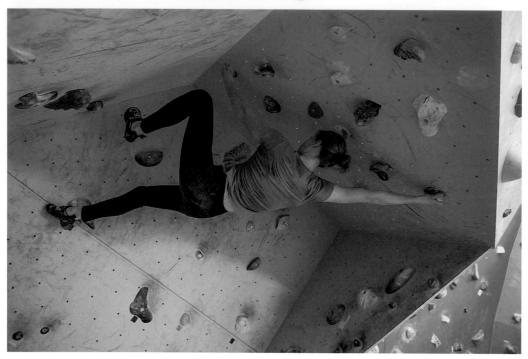

When clinging to a wall 40 feet in the air, you can't zone out. Reality turns into sweaty palms gripping climbing holds, feet searching for new places to land, and a lot of adrenaline. At least the ropes, harnesses, and belayers below prevent things from going wrong—if you fall off the wall, you've got a safety net.

When I first took a rock climbing class in college, I loved how it felt like chess on a wall, problem solving your way up a sheer cliff. But when I arrived at a local climbing gym for a

Climbing 101 class and saw the 45-foot walls speckled with colored holds and climbers moving up the walls like Spider-Man, I realized I had forgotten a critical component of climbing—height. The way forward is up.

Climbers are strong, and for good reason. The push, pull, and resistance of rock climbing builds strength, and one study showed that it is a major cardiovascular challenge for your body, with a big increase in heart rate and oxygen used, especially the more difficult the climb. One study also showed that eight weeks of bouldering—or harness-free climbing on boulders or boulder-height outcroppings—reduced the severity of depression.

My intro class was led by instructor Nick, who guides on Washington's 14,411-foot Mount Rainier. The 20-foot wall we were going to practice on didn't faze him whatsoever, but my stomach turned staring up at this relatively short climb.

Class started with a discussion on climbing gear, including harnesses, ropes, and carabiners, with Nick quizzing us to ensure we knew what to do to keep ourselves and our climbing partners safe. We learned to tie the rewoven figure eight used by climbers, how to set ourselves up to be belayed, and how to be the belayer and anchor point to keep another climber safe on the wall. He taught us partner checks, commands, and other technical details about climbing, all crucial to safe climbing.

Then he had us climb, and I discovered that the 20-foot wall was easier than it looked. In no time at all, I'd reached the top of an easy route. I felt proud and loved the view, even if it was of gray climbing walls.

Belaying someone else was more worrisome. I didn't know if a fellow student should put their life in my hands, even with Nick as backup on the belay. But to ensure we could do it well, he made us practice falls with no warning. It was a good exercise for me as a climber to trust someone would catch me. It was especially good practice for me as a belayer to make sure I stayed alert and could catch someone.

It was time to move on to the main part of the gym, with walls that were more than twice as high—about 45 feet. Gulp. Nick gave us a quick rundown on routes, from easy to difficult, and pointed out a couple of routes to work on.

Once I started climbing, the wall felt three times as high as the one we had just left. Not only did my legs tremble from the effort of balancing on tiny holds and my arms shake from pulling me up, but I could also feel fear-of-heights sweats coating my hands. I panicked a couple of times when I couldn't figure out the next hold to step on. I reminded myself to calm down, look around, and find another hold.

Top-rope climbing, tied into a rope anchored at the peak of the route, is the safest way to climb, Nick said, and a fear of heights is healthy. It will make you double-check your gear and focus on safety. You don't want to get overly confident when taking yourself this high up off the ground, he said. I would never call myself overconfident on a climbing wall, but the class bolstered my belief that I had enough skills to take a bouldering class.

At first glance, indoor bouldering looks a lot like indoor rock climbing. You need climbing shoes and chalk for your hands, and you scamper up routes with hand- and footholds set at varying degrees of challenge. Unlike rock climbing, you don't use a harness. The climbs are shorter. You can boulder solo at a gym; you don't need a belaying partner. On the flip side, if you boulder alone, you don't have a partner to celebrate your triumphs or call out advice on a challenging route. (Word to the wise: Don't boulder solo, particularly if you move outside. Boulder with a buddy.)

I went to a local bouldering gym to take the basics class. Our teacher, Chad, took us to a kids' party room to play around on an easy wall.

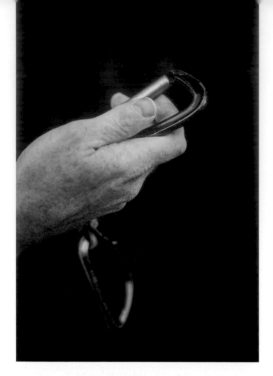

Chad emphasized the importance of warming up with jumping jacks or other cardio. Another simple way to warm up is to traverse a wall using holds, moving blood into your core, shoulders, hands, and legs.

Bouldering condenses the most technical parts of rock climbing into one little route, Chad told us, which made me realize it might be more complex than I'd thought. But I was determined—a quality I find critical when I'm afraid. Because make no mistake, fear hummed in my head as Chad gave us some chalk and sent us off.

Hoisting myself up the wall felt familiar. Some rock climbing techniques, like turning my body sideways to the wall to keep my hips close, came back from climbing class. I forgot to straighten my arms, to rely on my skeleton rather than muscles to preserve energy. Instead, I tried to muscle through. My forearms shook from the effort.

Chad advised us to stay on the balls of our feet, and he walked us through the names of different holds. All I could retain was that some holds are hard to grip and some are not.

Next, we practiced climbing the start of a route, then letting go and falling onto the thick mats. The pads in a bouldering gym are thicker than those at rock climbing gyms; learning to fall well is crucial when you don't have a harness.

Releasing myself from the wall was nerve-wracking; I didn't want to let go. But the technique is easy to do—drop onto the pads and let your legs roll up and back once you hit the floor to lessen the impact. I knew it was an essential skill, so I made myself practice until it felt more natural.

Growing into a better climber requires planning and strategy, Chad said. Start at the low end of the rating system with V0 or V1, and do all those climbs in a room first. Once you feel comfortable, move up to the next degree of difficulty. New routes are set all the time, so there will always be challenging routes at a gym. Good climbers practice all the time.

We climbed one route as a class and were then released to climb on our own. I tackled the low-level V1s with yellow holds. I thought I would be petrified without a harness, but I managed to stay focused. I was anxious close to the top but thrilled when I finished the routes, especially the harder ones.

Despite my nervousness, I pronounced bouldering fun to anyone who would listen, and I decided to go back for more technical instruction on how to climb well. My local gym, Bouldering Two, teaches foundational techniques for climbing. Our teacher, Adrian, talked about how to be as efficient as possible when moving from hold to hold. The cleaner and more intentional you are in the way you place your feet, adjust your hips, and

OR TRY . . . CLIMBING OUTDOORS

When I moved from climbing inside to outside, molded holds morphed into craggy granite, rough under my fingertips. The sounds of the gym melted away, replaced by the sound of birds chirping and my own breathing. My view shifted from a busy gym with bright-blue mats to a forest floor carpeted with pine needles and peekaboo views of snowcapped peaks. Climbing moved from a physical challenge of trying to work out a route to a full-sensory experience.

Moving outdoors is a huge shift in other ways, too. It requires additional preparation and more experience than climbing at a gym. Some gyms offer classes to help you transition outdoors; you also may have made some friends who are comfortable with outdoor climbing and can offer guidance on the best spots and the prep required.

Climbing outside means more investment in time and money, whether it's buying or renting bouldering crash pads or purchasing ropes and a backpack. You'll add in hiking time to get to prime spots, plus new challenges with longer routes. Your desire to become a better technical climber may explode once you realize you want to learn to lead climb on lengthier routes. You'll build endurance, and your love of climbing may become all-consuming.

As with any sport, it helps to start slowly. I have had experienced friends who have shown me the basics and guided me through. Climbing outside is a major shift in prep and mindset. Take on easier climbs for the experience before moving on to more advanced climbs. You'll make new friends and build an even deeper sense of camaraderie when you move your climbing or bouldering outside.

reach for the next hold, the less you will tire yourself out and the more interesting your climbing will become.

This is what I'm talking about.

Adrian's first topic, center of gravity, was the most important one, he said. If we could master this one principle, we would walk away better climbers. We practiced standing on the ground and shifting our center of gravity from one foot to the other, standing so firmly on one leg that we could lift the other easily. Balance? I've got balance dialed, I thought. Thank you, yoga.

The next topic, straight arms, was a technique I had not mastered. Adrian showed us how to step both feet onto holds and bend our legs into a squat position while gripping climbing holds with arms extended straight. This allows you to rely on strong, stable legs for endurance rather than upper body muscles that may be strong but tire out faster. I saw how to translate this theory to the real world, hanging off the wall in a squat, my elbows straight, feeling rather like a hobbit.

To learn weight transfer, we started in the deep, hobbit squat low on the wall, arms straight, and shifted our weight to one foot. Adrian then directed us to extend the other foot to a hold and then reach with one hand for another.

Holds naturally tell you which way to grab and how to position your body if you look at them strategically. Practice moving your weight in the natural direction for a hold, Adrian told us, and you will move more efficiently.

We worked on a mini-route to apply all our new techniques. It was a breeze when Adrian told us what to do, crossing arms from hold to hold, and reaching diagonally with one arm.

Then we added in twists, or what I think of as moving my hips closer to the wall. A twist makes the climb look and feel more effortless. The more you twist in toward the wall, the more you flow as you climb, Adrian said, demonstrating a balletic traverse. I want to climb like that, I thought.

For the first time, the techniques clicked. I knew certain techniques make things easier, like keeping hips close to the wall. But now, I had words and a pattern of moving for the beautiful, fluid climbing I often witnessed and could never incorporate into my own climbing. It was far easier when I followed routes Adrian mapped out. I had work to do to apply the technique on my own. But his progression—stabilize your center of gravity, transfer your weight, reach for a hold, and twist your hips to the wall—can be used for every move.

My brain was in excited overload. For the first time, I realized I could progress faster, using fewer moves up on harder routes, saving energy as I climbed. I could execute—or at least practice—more efficient climbing.

Climbing requires full-body effort, and I love that I now know how to conserve energy in the midst of an intense physical challenge. It is the pathway to getting stronger, taking on more challenging routes, and growing in my climbing.

GET STARTED INDOOR CLIMBING

Take an intro to climbing or bouldering class at a local climbing gym to get to know the equipment and how the gym setup works.

QUICK TIPS

- Use a chalk bag. You don't have to have one, but it helps to have chalk handy if you find your hands sweat at a certain height on the wall like mine do.
- Though climbing may appear to be primarily strength based, hip and shoulder mobility also make a difference as you progress up more advanced routes. Consider adding in a yoga practice to elevate your climbing skills.
- I was surprised by how much finger and hand strength I needed to build. Serious climbers use fingerboards with tiny holds to strengthen their fingers at the gym or at home. You also need to toughen up the skin on your hands, building layers of calluses to handle rough rock or climbing holds. Be patient; increasing tendon strength and toughening skin by climbing regularly takes time.

BEFORE YOU GO

Equipment: Climbing shoes, harness, chalk bag, stretchy clothes that you can move in.
Cost: An introduction to climbing at a gym costs $40 to $60 to learn the basics, from tying ropes to belay technique. This may or may not include membership costs, which can

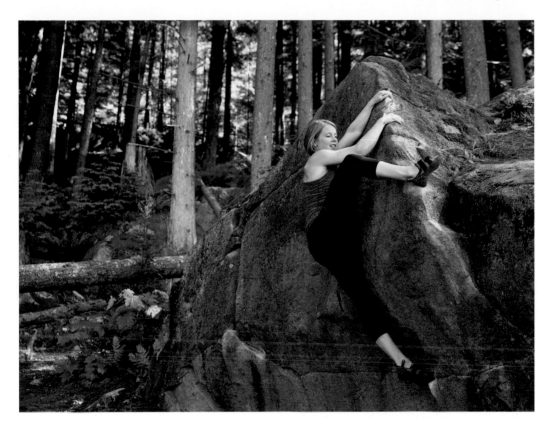

be charged per session or a monthly fee. In a city, the monthly fee ranges from $60 to $100.

CHALLENGE YOURSELF

Once you are comfortable with the equipment and basic climbs, climbing offers many layers of challenge to grow. Try these goals:

Level Up: Climb one additional day a week and complete all the gym's foundational climbs.

Reach Goal: Take a technique-oriented class and climb two additional days per week. Progress into higher difficulty ratings to challenge yourself with your climbs.

Adventure Goal: Plan a climbing or bouldering trip outdoors (see sidebar). Make sure to go with an instructor or friends who know how to climb outdoors, and be prepared with equipment, including ropes for climbing and crash pads for bouldering. Many gyms offer classes to prep you to move your climbing outside.

DISCOVERY: *Indoor Climbing*

	1ST	2ND	3RD
DATE			
DURATION			
RATING (1 TO 5 STARS)	★ ★ ★ ★ ★	★ ★ ★ ★ ★	★ ★ ★ ★ ★

What did you discover about your relationship with heights while climbing? Do you have a fear of heights? Did it stop you from climbing, or were you able to keep going?

What did you learn about the physical strength required for climbing? If rock climbing, what did you learn about working with another person and trusting them with your safety?

Did you have fun challenging yourself, or did you struggle to keep going when things got tough? How did you feel the first time you accomplished a route tougher than you thought you could do?

Month **8**

Roller Skating

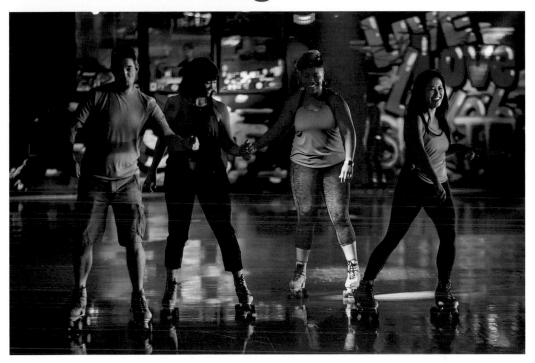

I have taken more beginner lessons in sports than I care to count, and yet there I was, realizing yet again a fundamental rule when taking up a new physical activity—get help.

My previous attempts at roller skating as an adult were on family outings, when I was looking for something fun and active for our family to do. I learned over several open skate sessions that skating forward on my own is possible, thanks to many years as an ice skater. But balance on roller skates is fundamentally more difficult with a kid hanging on. Stopping is nearly impossible, kid or no kid. That's what walls are for, right?

But in one hour at a local skating rink, roller skating instructors taught me to stop both forward and backward and added in crossovers so I could skate in circles. I learned to turn backward and keep skating, then practiced turning forward while still moving. For good measure, they had me practice a derby start and a derby stop, which I hadn't heard of before class.

Take a lesson. Trust me.

Roller skating is considered an aerobic fitness sport by the American Heart Association. I'll vouch that it requires a lot of balance and core strength to stay upright! It also is a low-impact sport, and if you challenge yourself with speed and technique, it becomes an even more fun and physical activity to take on.

At a regular weekend class, I was pleasantly surprised to find three instructors working with a range of skill sets, from total newbie to more advanced. I started with the beginners, where Alex taught us to walk forward with skates in a V-shape. What do you do if you're about to fall? The rule is: "Oh no,

OR TRY . . . ICE SKATING

For most of my adult life, I took my childhood ice skating lessons for granted. I'm glad I can stand on two feet on the ice without toppling over. Jumps and spins are cool party tricks. I love flying across the ice and feeling cold air rush past my face. But I'm rarely nostalgic for the years I spent practicing spins and jumps, doing drill team practice, or putting on sparkly outfits with twirly skirts.

Then I took an adult ice skating class. I left thinking that every parent needs to put their child on ice skates, stat. Get your balance down early, and you'll have it for the rest of your life.

Our adult basics class included a lot of moms picking up skating for the first time while their kids took lessons. Our teacher, Susie, showed us how to skate forward, balance on one foot, swizzle, and skate backward—all foundational skating skills.

I decided to stay on for a more advanced class, where the steps grew more complicated. We worked on dance steps, three-turns, and brackets, which required turning from an outside edge to an inside edge. Suzie spotted what threw someone off balance, whether a hip thrust in the wrong direction or limp arms, and helped them correct their technique.

Afterward, I joined in for the free skate; I wanted to see what else I could remember. Basic jumps like toe loops and salchows came back easily. I could still do a fast scratch spin.

Ice arenas haven't changed that much since I was a kid. During free skate, kids flopped on their bellies to slide across the ice while a little figure skater practiced a sit spin. As I circled the rink, listening to the thwack of hockey sticks at an adjacent rink and inhaling sharp, cold air, I got nostalgic. I was transported to the days of aching feet, snacks of soft pretzels with cheese, and running around an ice arena wearing tight braids and makeup.

The adult lessons reminded me that those early years skating were worth it. Lessons trained the clumsy out of my feet and taught me balance that still serves me today. Competing taught me discipline and practice at a young age, and that muscle memory isn't theoretical.

Take lessons young, and ice skating will never leave you. Take ice skating up as an adult to remind yourself you can learn new skills—and improve balance—at any age.

go low!" Alex told me and the kids. Put your hands on your knees when a fall is imminent.

After Alex watched me V-step, I graduated to another teacher, Shaun. I told him I needed to learn to stop, and he showed me a lunge, dragging my back skate's rubber stopper on the wood floor to slow down. It was so straightforward that I nearly smacked myself on the forehead. How did I not figure this one out on my own?

Shaun showed me that the key to turning backward is to skate forward on one foot and then do a quick turn onto the other foot. It was easier said than done, especially since skating backward was a slow adventure.

We also worked on crossovers, tracing painted circles in the middle of the rink. You put all your weight on one foot, then lift the other foot over. Balancing on one foot at a time is an essential skating skill, but one I was reluctant to practice for fear of crashing. The hard, wood floor looked painful.

Shaun left me to practice, and I flashed back to my childhood ice skating days, practicing technique alone. I did a big, swooping figure eight, working on crossovers on my right side then switching to the awkward left. I practiced my stops.

Once crossovers felt more comfortable, I tried to transition from skating forward to backward. This was scary, and not so smooth. Shaun said it takes 20 hours of practice to get comfortable at any of the skills I was learning.

I was sweating by now, though whether from fear of falling or effort, it was hard to know. I finally did enough turns to feel semi-comfortable. Shaun, who had been helping others, came back and had me work on my backward skating, starting with reverse swizzles. I brought my feet together, moved them out in a half moon shape, and then pulled them back together, stringing several together. I started to get some momentum but not too much.

Shaun told me I wasn't falling enough. Let me clarify: I hadn't fallen at all. You should fall at least three times during the class, then we'll know you're out of your comfort zone, he pronounced, as kids crashed around me. They had no issue with the hard, wood floor.

Was I being a perfectionist? Was I afraid? Was I all of the above?

I frowned then went at the new skills with more vigor. I practiced turning backward on the other, less comfortable side. I swizzled backward and went faster, then tried stopping backward.

Alex spotted me and came over to explain that roller skates are made for backward stops, with the rubber stopper in front. For my backward stop, I scissored my feet, right foot slightly ahead of the left, and then dragged one rubber stop so I could slow without falling on my face. He demonstrated the derby stop, putting both stoppers down at the same time, heels in the air. The derby stop calls for wild arm flair, by the way. We had ventured into not-at-all comfortable and highly-likely-to-fall territory, a.k.a. my potential freak-out zone.

Shaun introduced one more transition, swiveling both feet at the same time 180 degrees to turn around quickly and skate backward. He showed me a derby start, which looks like a derby stop; feet scissored, heels up and toes down, balanced up on the stoppers. It gives you the traction to bolt at the start of your skate.

What if you don't want to skate fast? (I didn't say this out loud. But I thought it. I thought it loudly.)

Shaun gave me my last challenge—do a derby start balanced on my rubber stoppers, run a couple steps, skate, swivel backward, derby stop.

Yikes.

Despite my inner busybody shouting that this was all a terrible idea, I decided to push myself. I did what Shaun instructed, derby start to derby stop. It was not pretty, nor stable, but I did it. I didn't fall, which mattered to me, and probably proved to my teachers I was still holding back. But I didn't care. I was tuckered out.

Like all sports, roller skating requires you to learn a few key skills, a worthwhile effort since skating can be so much fun. I advise going in with an attitude that you'll love it. My favorite parts of skating are grooving to the music at a family skate, swiveling my feet, and enjoying the chaos of skating around wipeouts. I always dance to "The Hokey Pokey" when it comes on. You'll get to know the standard songs at your local rink the more you go.

My advice? Take a lesson or two. You may be surprised by what you learn, and on the next family outing, you'll definitely have more fun.

GET STARTED ROLLER SKATING

Take an intro lesson at a local rink, getting comfortable with skating forward and learning how to stop without using a wall (although the wall remains a convenient option).

QUICK TIPS

- Wear comfortable clothing to skate, but it's also a time you could go retro, put on some neon, and sweep your hair into a side ponytail. Just sayin'.
- If you're serious about skating, look into buying your own skates. Rentals can only take you so far if you want to increase your skating skills.

BEFORE YOU GO

Equipment: Roller skates, comfortable clothes, and a fun attitude.

Cost: Skate rental and rink time are typically $10 to $20. Some rinks include the skate rental with your entrance fee.

CHALLENGE YOURSELF

Once you've learned to skate forward and stop, ramp up the fun at your skating sessions with these tricks.

Level Up: Add one additional skate per week to practice what you learned from the intro class and work on crossovers.

Reach Goal: Sign up for a regular series of skating lessons to learn more challenging moves, like skating backward or the transition from forward skating to backward.

Adventure Goal: Does your town have roller derby? Now that's an adventure. Your derby league may teach the fundamentals of skating and roller derby. Get yourself some new skates and learn what it takes to peel around a rink at top speed!

DISCOVERY: *Roller Skating*

	1ST	2ND	3RD
DATE			
DURATION			
RATING (1 TO 5 STARS)	★ ★ ★ ★ ★	★ ★ ★ ★ ★	★ ★ ★ ★ ★

When was the last time you went roller skating? What was different from what you remembered?

What did you find the most challenging about putting four wheels on each foot? Were you worried about falling, looking silly, or not being able to keep up?

When you skated for the second time, what did you notice that changed from the first time you skated? Were you able to have more control or be more playful? What did you enjoy about skating?

What new skills did you learn from roller skating? What skills would you like to learn the next time you go?

Zumba

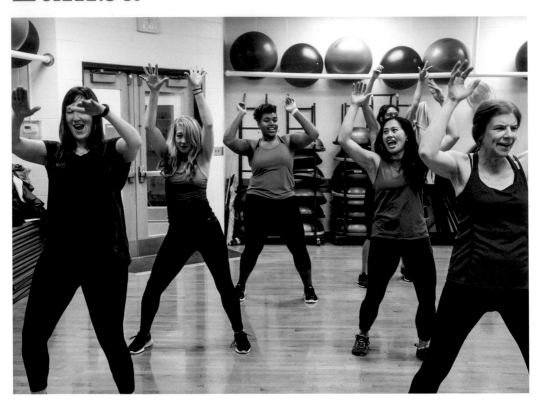

I hadn't thought through the ramifications of taking Zumba at 7:00 a.m.—not beyond putting it on my calendar and setting an alarm the night before to be sure I got ready in time to drive in darkness to the gym. I am not only not perky at that hour, without coffee, I am barely awake. I realized my mistake on my way to the class. It was already too late to snag a cup of joe.

When I arrived at the brightly lit fitness room, women were milling around chatting before class began; they appeared energized, or at least alert. I chalked it up to a smarter morning strategy. They must have had coffee, I mused. There's no other explanation for being able to talk at this hour.

I cringed a little inside when we all faced a large, mirrored wall and the loud, cheerful music began. If teacher Lilo had issues with the early hour, she masked it well. As soon as the music started, she was at the front of the room, smiling at us and moving side to side, encouraging us to get our bodies warmed up.

It was join or be left in the dust by the regulars. In my non-caffeinated haze, I observed that they already seemed to know the songs and the steps Lilo demonstrated. I was not off to a good start. But I have one essential idiosyncrasy that made the difference—I am willing to throw myself into whatever I am being asked to do in a class, no matter how silly it makes me feel. I soon found myself relying on this quirk.

With a mix of dance moves and nonstop movement, Zumba has become a popular workout. It makes moving easy and fun with simple, accessible dance steps choreographed to lively Latin music, though Zumba classes also include hip-hop and other popular music.

Moving to music boosts your mood and self-confidence, and it reduces stress. It also challenges coordination and balance. Even simple choreography shifts your brain to focus more and improve your memory. Zumba also brings the cardio, with nonstop songs and choreography that keep your heart rate up throughout the class. The motto: just keep dancing.

A Zumba class can be vigorous and high energy, with a lot of jumping and energetic arm movements. You also can make it low impact as needed, stepping side to side instead of bouncing, and keeping your arms next to you to tamp down the level of effort. You can move in a lot of new ways without straining joints or being hard on your body, which makes it ideal for any age.

You get a huge variety of Latin dance in a Zumba class, which is an excellent education in dance steps. I was familiar with the merengue and salsa steps, and there were also cumbia, reggaeton, flamenco, and bachata. Lilo did each step slowly and with exaggerated movements through the first count and then sped up to match the beat of the song, so I found the choreography easy to follow, even with unfamiliar steps.

I soon realized Lilo had signals for what we did with our feet and arms for each dance. She held up two fingers when we doubled up on moves or spun a finger to indicate it was time to repeat the series of steps we had just done. Though I didn't always catch her signals, the moves and structure of the class were sinking in.

At the beginning, I felt anxious about getting steps wrong, especially considering everyone around me seemed to have the footwork memorized. I realized I would have more fun if I just let myself get into the beat. I still messed up steps, but as long as I kept moving, I could get back on track.

Soon, I got over my early morning resistance. I shook my shoulders and bumped my hips with the regulars, who smiled and hooted as we danced. I loved watching them anticipate every shimmy of their shoulders or spin side to side. They knew most of the songs and steps, but they told me Lilo throws in a couple new ones every week for a challenge.

I started to smile, especially when Lilo instructed us do some pelvic swivels then playfully covered her eyes when we exaggerated the swirl of our hips.

Most of the music was Latin, but we also danced to Top 40 hits. Lilo whipped out red,

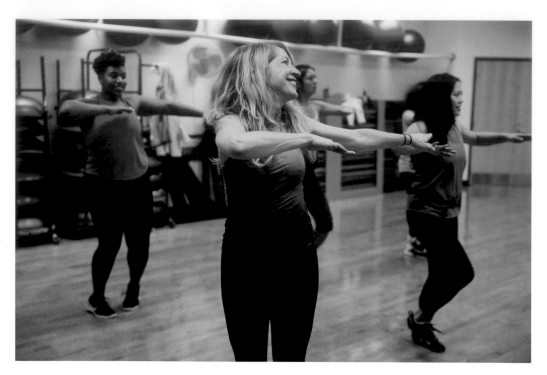

purple, and green coin-covered hip scarves for a Bollywood song so we could work on some belly dance skills. We each grabbed one and tied it around our hips. I liked my scarf's jingling coins, and we merrily thrust our hips side to side and tried to imitate Lilo's emphatic bumps and swivels.

Throughout the class, the dance moves were relatively simple and low impact, doing easy box steps or grapevines side to side. You had the option of making each move more animated, with deeper squats or adding knee lifts or a hop to increase the impact. I waved my arms overhead, dipped low, and shimmied as best I could.

Lilo kept the energy up throughout the hour, encouraging us to keep going and have fun as my face grew shiny from effort and sweat dripped down my back. By the last few minutes of class, I was grateful for a couple of slow songs for stretching after all the vigorous dance steps.

When class was over, I felt energized and ready for the day.

Zumba has become a popular alternative to aerobics classes, and I can see its appeal. I know people who take Zumba several times a week as their main way to move, de-stress, and bring energy and fun back into their day. Zumba teachers must be licensed, but they are free to choose their own combinations of songs and choreography as long as class is consistently 70 percent Latin or international rhythms, and I've met folks who make it a point to follow their favorite teachers because of their unique styles.

Take Zumba early in the day, and you might not even need your morning cup of coffee.

GET STARTED WITH ZUMBA

If you're looking for a way to have fun while getting exercise, and you're ready to loosen up a bit through dance, take a Zumba class once a week.

QUICK TIPS

- If you belong to a gym, they likely have Zumba on the fitness class calendar. If not, check with your local community center to see if classes are offered.
- The class is energetic; remember that you can always modify or reduce its intensity.

BEFORE YOU GO

Equipment: Wear sneakers and clothes to sweat in. Bring some water.

Cost: If you have a gym membership, Zumba may be included. Studios and community centers frequently offer Zumba, with class prices averaging around $10 in a city.

CHALLENGE YOURSELF

Once you've gotten comfortable swaying your hips and following a teacher, it's easy to get more Zumba in your life. Here are ways to step it up:

Level Up: After you've taken one class, add it in twice a week. Even if you already have other movement activities you enjoy, bring this in to mix up the energy and make workouts more fun.

Reach Goal: Ramp up the energy by tackling the higher-impact components of class, from using your arms to bouncing or jumping if your joints allow.

Adventure Goal: If you're really enjoying class, branch out to new teachers and see what you can learn from different instructors and their styles.

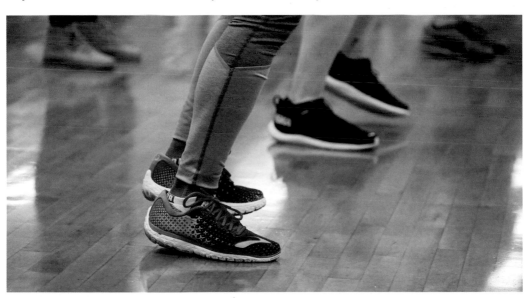

DISCOVERY: *Zumba*

	1ST	2ND	3RD
DATE			
DURATION			
RATING (1 TO 5 STARS)	★ ★ ★ ★ ★	★ ★ ★ ★ ★	★ ★ ★ ★ ★

What did you expect from taking a Zumba class? Did it live up to your expectations, or were you surprised by what you experienced?

How did dancing make you feel?

What did you discover about moving your body in a dance class compared to how you normally move?

What kind of dance steps did you pick up that you didn't know before Zumba?

Month **9**

Biking

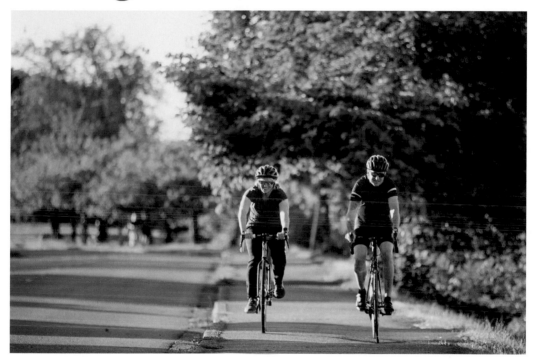

Whenever I have changed homes, my bicycle has moved with me, typically from a shed to a garage, depending on the house. I bought the bike with a great intention—to ride it. At the time, I lived near an easy cycling road that shut down on Sundays in summer specifically for biking access.

I also had visions of becoming a bike commuter, a person who skips driving to ride a bike everywhere. I would cut back on time in my car, helping to save money and the environment. I was excited at the beginning and went out once or twice, but as soon as temperatures dropped and rain came, the bike stayed indoors.

I've gone on long rides, encouraged by cyclist friends, and I even rode along an interstate (on the cycling path), a mildly terrifying and deafening experience. I survived an 18-mile ride that required extra gear, including a tire-changing kit and a water bottle setup. I reasoned that it was an investment

OR TRY . . . INDOOR CYCLING

People have loved indoor cycling for what feels like ages. I started going to get into cycling shape. Then I discovered the masochistic side of me enjoys getting yelled at (lovingly) by cycling instructors.

I went to a national chain's nearby location. The place was slick, with high ceilings, towels, and clip-in shoes as part of its high-flying prices.

They shut the lights off once class starts. A leaderboard occasionally flashes everyone's stats when the teacher decides to motivate you for mini-bursts. The music is so loud, they offer earplugs. But if you get the right teacher, it's also hugely fun. I liked cycling in the dark with my teacher shouting, "Challenge is change!" to keep me focused and cycling hard.

Our teacher pushed us to high levels of resistance, and we also did a lot of racing at low resistance. My legs burned, but my knees never felt taxed.

But then the weighted bars came out for tricep and bicep exercises. There was a two-pound bar and a four-pound bar—or combined for six pounds. I went with four pounds because after cycling for 28 minutes, my legs were already burning, I was dripping sweat, and arm weights were the last thing I wanted to do.

Right after the weighted bars, our teacher snapped off the leaderboard. I had a brief flash of annoyance that I could no longer obsess over rankings, then decided I'd just keep cycling faster to try to catch up to the leader.

The next time the leaderboard flashed, I had fallen farther behind. I changed my focus to my own performance, seeing if I could reach my own goal. I just missed it, but I know I can push a little harder next time.

for future rides. But after feeling proud of my efforts, I stashed my bike and gear at home and forgot about it.

Riding a bike is excellent exercise, and I have friends who have taken on the challenge of a century (100-mile) ride. Bikes also serve as great transportation. Cycling is a low-impact choice to get your heart rate up and your blood pumping while also strengthening your legs and core. If you're not interested in cycling for exercise, it is quicker than walking or sometimes even taking transit to get somewhere, with less environmental impact than a car. Over short distances where traffic is bad, it can be faster than driving—and you don't have to hunt for a parking space.

Despite the benefits, if asked about biking, for transportation in particular, I had excuses. I drove a lot between places for work, and riding a bike was slower. I lived on a hill. Bodies of water lie between me and the places I need to go. I don't like riding in the rain. Clearly, I wasn't going to start riding on my own. I needed help.

I found Anne and her husband, Tim, who run a business dedicated to working with people on cycling logistics. Anne meets a lot of non-riders like me. Many people would like to commute to work by bicycle, but

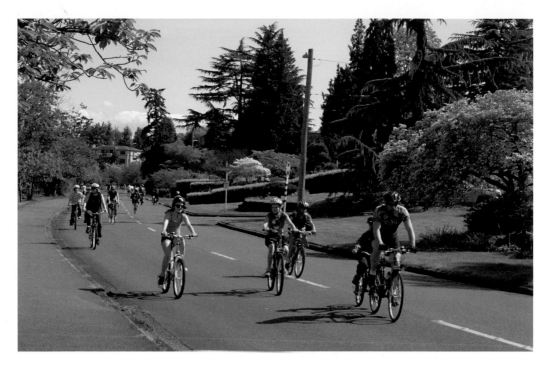

everything from gear to finding the best route prevents them from acting on riding. I knew I was capable of working this out on my own, but my commitment to follow through was lacking. Once I watched Tim, a certified bike mechanic, tune up my bike and looked at the route Anne researched for me, I was happy I'd farmed out the work to experts.

Commuting by bike doesn't work for me most days because I don't have a regular work commute. I lead a nomadic life, driving to different appointments or classes each day. Anne suggested adding cycling to other parts of my life, like riding to the grocery store that was less than a mile away from my home. It was such an obvious suggestion, I felt dense for not thinking of it myself. I also lived near a water taxi service that goes directly to downtown Seattle. I'd never ridden to downtown

because I was intimidated by a large, high-speed arterial bridge. Anne said she could come up with a solution that allowed me to skirt the bridge and would help me with the final push up the hill to my home. Sold.

Tim did the bike tune-up first, recommending fenders to prevent water from splashing on my legs and adding a rack to transport groceries. After he pumped up my tires and checked out a rattle, he called my bike good to go. Anne and I set a route: we'd cruise down to the water taxi and circle back up to my regular grocery store. It sounded easy enough, though maybe I should have been more wary of the hill climb.

Before we left, Anne went over the rules of the road. Some I knew, like keep an eye on parked cars; cyclists must watch out for a sudden car door opening that could cause serious injury if you hit it. I didn't know it was legal to ride on sidewalks in my city, though pedestrians have the right of way.

The downhill ride to the water taxi was easy, with Anne noting potholes and other perils as we rode. At the water taxi stand, rather than ride over to downtown Seattle, she showed me how to lock my bike properly, making sure to get both the body of the bike and a tire secured, for when I did make the trip.

For the ride to the nearby grocery store, rather than going back up the steep hill we'd cruised down, Anne had researched another route on a longer road with a gentler grade—or so she thought.

We rode over a flat road first then turned off to head up the hill. At the start, things

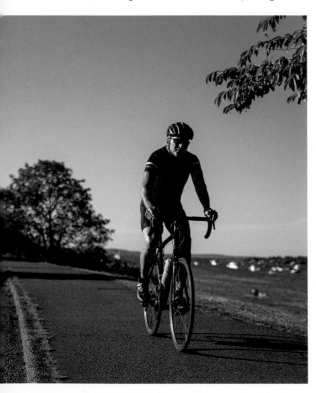

were fine. I set my gear to the lowest level so I had less resistance from my pedals as I climbed up the hill. We chatted a bit along the way, enjoying the beautiful road and weaving up through a greenbelt with trees lining the street and green foliage providing cover and filtered light. But as we rode, I realized the upward incline wasn't leveling out and that the ride might get harder. My legs started to tire out, even with my gear at the lowest setting. I saved my breath, and we stopped talking.

Anne told me the two biggest challenges for cyclists in Seattle are hills and traffic; if you live in a flat city, for biking reasons, I envy you. We faced no traffic, but the hill was getting the best of me. Anne said there was no shame in getting off a bike and walking. For the last push, I might have made it, but my legs burned. I decided to check my pride and told Anne I wanted to walk. We hopped off our bikes for the final steep slope of the hill before getting back on them again. We rode over to the grocery store and then circled back to my house on a flat road.

Most of the cyclists I know are hard-core—they do epic road races or mountain bike every weekend, using their bikes for an intense thrill. That's an excellent, fun reason to bike. If you're like me, however, and you're not in for an adrenaline rush, it's helpful to remember how versatile a bike can be. When left to my own devices, my habit is to get in a car for transportation. If I have time, I walk. Now, I realize all I need to do to break those patterns is to go to the shed and get my bike. That might even prompt me to venture on longer rides, just for fun and to move more. First, though, my bike needs another tune-up.

GET STARTED BIKING

Pick a destination close to where you live for your first ride—maybe a coffee shop, the library, or a grocery store. Give yourself a solid chunk of time to ride the route so you can get to know the streets and traffic patterns. Or find a bike path and just explore. Local biking groups or clubs are also great resources, with guided beginner rides and support for new riders.

QUICK TIPS

- You don't need professional help to map out a bike commute route, though it sure is nice! You can use Google Maps to figure out a route; test-ride the route first, without time pressure, so you know how long it takes.
- If you need a bike, look for a local bike shop to rent a bike or try out a few before you buy.
- Get your bike tuned up before you set out on a ride for the first time, especially if your bike has been sitting around for a year or three, and pick up the tools you'll need in case you get a flat. Or find a class at a local bike shop or watch videos online to learn to fix a flat and do other basic bike maintenance.

BEFORE YOU GO

Equipment: Bike, helmet, clip-on shoes if you have clip-on pedals, tools for repairing a flat tire, bike lock, sweat-wicking layers.
Cost: A daylong bike rental costs between $30 and $65 per day, depending on the style of bike. Most rentals come with a helmet, bike lock, and may also include a flat tire repair kit.

CHALLENGE YOURSELF

Once you've gotten yourself on your bike on a regular basis, the options to challenge yourself open up. Try these:

Level Up: Map your ride to work and do a run on the weekend to see if it's something you can build into your schedule.
Reach Goal: Start commuting to work one or two days a week or use your bike for a regular errand, like going to the grocery store or the library.
Adventure Goal: Do a longer ride for fun. Take on a two- to three-hour ride on a weekend. See what new trails, roads, and sights you experience that you otherwise miss when driving a car. Local biking clubs also host longer rides; look into joining a group for an extended outing.

DISCOVERY: *Biking*

	1ST	2ND	3RD
DATE			
DURATION			
RATING (1 TO 5 STARS)	★ ★ ★ ★ ★	★ ★ ★ ★ ★	★ ★ ★ ★ ★

Do you think of a bike as something to use for exercise or as a way to get around? If you've ridden or had a bike before, what way did you use it most?

Do you have a favorite childhood memory about riding a bike? What do you remember specifically about riding a bike as a kid?

What did you learn about your neighborhood or city from biking? What did you see that you hadn't noticed before? Did you become more aware of topographical elements, like hills, that had escaped your notice?

What did you learn about your physical conditioning from biking? Were you challenged by the ride?

RECOVERY: *Acupuncture*

My journey with acupuncture started with a shoulder ache that became intolerable. A friend at work raved about seeing an acupuncturist, so I made an appointment.

I lay facedown on the table as the acupuncturist placed needles all along my shoulder. He placed a heat lamp over the needles, and I melted under its warmth. He was the first person who told me to use heat to move stuck energy when injured. Only use ice within the first 24 hours of an injury, he said. It's advice I still use today. After three weeks of twice-weekly sessions, my shoulder pain disappeared.

Acupuncture is an ancient Chinese medicine used to treat hundreds of ailments. Fine needles are inserted at various acupressure points on the body. Research has shown it can help resolve pain and improve sleep and digestion. Traditionally, it's a practice to bring your body's energy flow back into balance.

I returned to acupuncture a few years later. I wanted to aid my recovery any way possible. At the very least, the twisting pain went down a notch after getting needles in my back and resting under the heat lamp.

After the injury healed, I went back to help recover from a surgery and I haven't stopped since. It has become a time for me to recover from pushing my body, a part of my own self-care, and a time to treat my body well.

One benefit of regular acupuncture is the opportunity to wind down into the parasympathetic state, when your breathing and heart rate slow and your body goes into rest mode. You put your phone aside and soften for 30 minutes or more. I almost always fall asleep.

At my sessions, I tell my acupuncturist what's been happening in my body, from the twinge in my foot to the persistent ache in my hip. I share what else is going on in my life, including work or family stress. I tell her if I feel a cold is coming on.

Once I'm on the table, my acupuncturist feels my foot, my hip, or gently presses on my belly. She looks at my tongue and takes my wrist to measure my pulse.

Then come the needles, set into familiar places, like my hip or over my surgical scar. Sometimes, they go in my neck or between my eyebrows.

Finally, I get my beloved heat lamp. Then I relax.

Most of the time, I barely feel needles going in, with just the occasional prick of sensation. When I need more intense work, I get deeper needling done; I sometimes leave those sessions sore but with my body ultimately restored.

Whether used to help heal an injury or imbalance, or as part of routine self-care, acupuncture has become an essential tool in caring for my physical and mental well-being.

Month **10**

Stair Walking

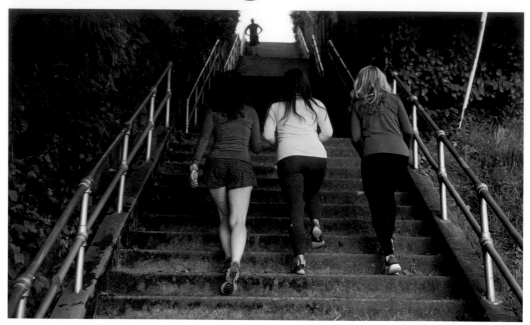

Walking by myself is pleasant, as far as movement goes, but if given the choice, I prefer the company of others, from strolling with my pup to catching up with friends. In fact, my friends and I even have a name for these jaunts: walk 'n' talks. It's the best way to share what's happening in our lives and get in some fresh air and good, vigorous movement at the same time.

Stair walks are especially fun. They're so popular in hilly Seattle that there are websites and books that share various maps with plenty of routes.

Queen Anne is perfect for a stair walk. It's one of the city's oldest—and steepest—neighborhoods. The neighborhood is built around one tall hill, which is about 450 feet high and crisscrossed by stairs. I chose a walk up the western side of Queen Anne Hill, where the streets are famously impassable by car in the icy winter and excellent for sledding during rare snowfalls.

I ended up walking alone, so I thought it was a good time to call my mom and catch up. But I soon realized a stair walk was not ideal for talking. My mom asked, "What are you doing?" as I huffed my way up and down the stairs and panted into my headset. I underestimated the effort needed to propel myself up stairs, and talking took away precious—and much needed—oxygen. A walk 'n' talk was only going to work with someone else next to me, huffing just as much. I ended the call and focused on the stairs.

Then I faced a logistical challenge—keeping track of my route. I'd picked a four-mile path from a website that offered directions for multiple stair walks with maps. The route zigged and zagged up and down small streets that didn't appear to be sending me in any particular direction. Then I realized my route wasn't about getting somewhere; it was about stairs, narrow and wide, steep and shallow, some with grand views of glistening water framed by mountains, others canopied by trees overhead. Sometimes, a flight of stairs was short, moving me up between streets; some flights were long and took me into what felt like people's backyards. It takes all types of stairs to get you up and down a steep hill in the city.

I started at a brisk pace but soon slowed down when I realized how steep the walk was. My legs and glutes burned as I climbed. I was happy when I arrived at flatter streets and was even more thrilled to head downhill, giving me a chance to catch my breath.

Many chunks of my walk offered panoramic views of Elliott Bay, cargo ships, and the snowcapped peaks of the Olympic Peninsula along with the Space Needle and the downtown core. These were the kind of classic Seattle views I wished I could share with a friend. I paused often to look around.

Another section of my walk took me to a beautiful piece of architecture known as

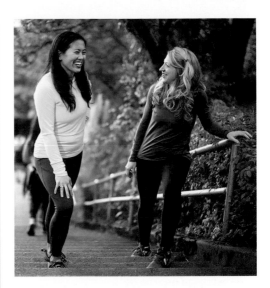

the Wilcox Wall—a tall retaining wall with a diamond pattern, archways, and grand street lamps framing a stairway. It's tucked away into the side of the hill, and you might not know it's there unless you live nearby.

Because I was walking on one of the first bluebird days of spring, there were flowers blooming everywhere. A light breeze cooled me off from the effort. The sky was a deep, vivid blue. It was a lovely afternoon to be outside, and I appreciated all that I saw. My stair walk took me down dead ends I wouldn't see while driving, dropped me into charming cul-de-sacs, and led me past beautiful old houses. I loved exploring the neighborhood and saw many other folks out for walks, though most weren't taking all the stairs like I was.

I ended up cutting my walk to about three miles, though not by choice—I was confused about where to go next. The good thing about Queen Anne is there is almost always another set of stairs nearby that you can take. I used Google Maps to route myself back to another section of the walk.

After about 45 minutes, I was tired and also happy I had not walked the full four-mile route. I checked my phone, which was tracking my progress: I had walked 6,000 steps and climbed the equivalent of 43 floors. I'll take it, I thought.

Walking is one of my everyday movement activities. I also turn to walking on active rest days, necessary as a break if I've been pushing my body on high-activity days. Walking stairs is perfect for an active rest day when I need to recover or if I'm looking for a more intense walk but don't want to stress my body. It's also ideal on the road; do a little research to find some stairs to add to a walk, and then head out the door.

Whether you're someone who walks frequently and would like to increase the intensity, or if you need to take your activity down a notch for a day, a stair walk is a lively way to challenge yourself. Walking itself has incredible benefits, from reducing the risk of developing breast cancer to preventing arthritis from forming; it also improves memory and brain function and helps maintain bone density. Add in stairs, and you'll layer in even more leg and glute strength work.

If you need additional motivation to go for a walk with the added oomph of stairs, snag a buddy to go with you. You can huff and puff your way to more energy and fun together.

GET STARTED STAIR WALKING

Go for a 30-minute walk that includes a few sets of stairs. Do it once a week.

QUICK TIPS

- You can usually find stairs, even if you're not in a hilly place. Walk up and down stairs in a building or at a mall. Find a park that spans multiple levels, and use the stairs. Go to a stadium and walk the stairs.
- Don't underestimate the challenge of stairs! Take breaks as needed.
- Substitute hills for stairs to mix up the terrain you're walking on. An incline of any kind adds challenge.
- Carry some water, especially if you're out on a hot day. You might be surprised by how thirsty you get and how tired you are by the end.

BEFORE YOU GO

Equipment: Sneakers or other comfortable shoes, clothes to sweat in.
Cost: Free.

CHALLENGE YOURSELF

As you get stronger, add in more challenge by extending your stair walks. Aim for these milestones:

Level Up: Take on a 30- to 45-minute walk that is at least half stairs, finding a way to keep moving up and down stairs during the walk, and do it once or twice a week.
Reach Goal: Lengthen your walk to one hour, with at least half of the route made up of stairs. See if you can find longer, steeper stairs to build into the walk.
Adventure Goal: Challenge yourself to plan out a two-hour walk that includes multiple sets of stairs throughout the route.

DISCOVERY: *Stair Walking*

	1ST	2ND	3RD
DATE			
DURATION			
RATING (1 TO 5 STARS)	★ ★ ★ ★ ★	★ ★ ★ ★ ★	★ ★ ★ ★ ★

What did you discover about the physical effort required to climb stairs? Were you surprised by the challenge, or did you find it easier than you imagined?

What did you learn about where you live from looking for stairs and walking them?

What was the best part of your stair walk, whether it was a view or overcoming a physical challenge?

What did you find the most challenging about a stair walk?

Month **10**

Tabata

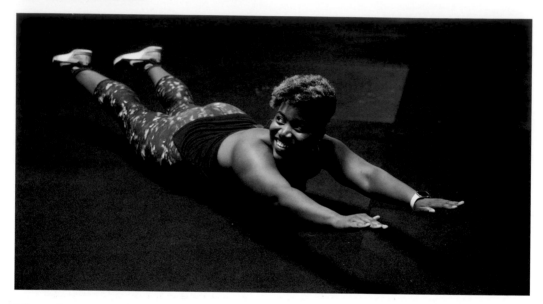

When I first heard about Tabata, which is a high-intensity interval training (HIIT) method, it sounded moderately tough but nothing I couldn't handle. Then I tried it, both with weights and one time using just body weight for the workout, maxing out pull-ups, sit-ups, push-ups, and squats for 20 seconds at a time.

Conclusion: Tabata does not rank in my Top 10 Ways to Work Out—unless I want a fierce and effective workout. Tabata boosts both aerobic and anaerobic fitness, which builds strength, speed, and power, and it does so in a short period of time. Sometimes, even I need something short and intense.

But do I want to do it? That's a different matter altogether.

Tabata—named for scientist Izumi Tabata, who studied the impact of high-intensity interval training on athletcs—calls for doing an exercise in intervals of 20 seconds on, 10 seconds off, for a total of eight rounds, which doesn't sound that bad. Tabata also includes a one-minute rest after a full round of eight is complete, and then you move on to a new exercise. Do five exercises or so, and you can get a complete workout in 25 minutes.

Although I knew I could do Tabata on my own, I wanted to explore other approaches to the workout. When I found a Total Body

Tabata class at a local gym that lasted longer than the usual 25 minutes, I couldn't tell if it would be better or worse than doing it on my own.

The class was packed. People clearly liked this method, and I hoped I would, too. We set up for class with stepper platforms, hand weights, stretchy bands, and square felt pieces for what I figured would be core work.

This Tabata class used the timing system as its foundation, staying with the 20-second bursts over four-minute rounds, and built onto it by throwing in cardio along with weight training. The class started off with a surge of loud music and an energetic warm-up, and then we dove in. For each round, we alternated two rounds of weight work with two rounds of cardio, then repeated it. Each round targeted different parts of the body, such as the shoulders, upper back, and core, mixed in with cardio such as lunges, burpees, and squats.

BODYWEIGHT EXERCISES FOR TABATA

Need some ideas for bodyweight exercises to get going on your Tabata workout? Use these five exercises as a baseline, building to a 25-minute workout. Make sure you warm up for five minutes before you start.

SQUATS: For squat form, start with your feet shoulder-width apart, lower your hips behind you and bring them below your knees. Do as many as you can for each 20-second interval. *Modification:* If you have trouble squatting with your heels down or feet parallel, turn your toes out, widen your stance, or fold a blanket or towel under your heels to build up to a full squat.

PLANKS: Start on your hands and knees. Plant your hands directly under your shoulders, straighten your legs, and come into a plank for a hold. Push down into the floor to engage the muscles in your upper back. Squeeze your quad muscles. Keep your head lifted so your neck is in line with the rest of your spine, and and make sure your hips stay level with your shoulders. Hold for 20 seconds. *Modification:* Bring your knees to the floor.

PUSH-UPS: Start in a strong plank position, then lower to the floor, pulling your elbows in toward your ribs. Press back up to a full plank with your core engaged. Do as many push-ups as you can in the 20-second time frame. *Modification:* Bring your knees to the ground or put your hands on a higher surface, like a coffee table or a wall, to lessen the intensity.

HOLLOW BODY: Lie down on your back. Lift your legs and your shoulders off the floor and extend your arms above your head. Rock back and forth for 20 seconds. *Modification:* Bring your knees into your chest and rock.

SUPERMAN: Lie down on your belly. Reach your arms forward like you are flying. Lift your chest and legs off the floor, squeezing your quad muscles and engaging your upper back. Hold this position for 20 seconds. *Modification:* Bring your arms back by your hips.

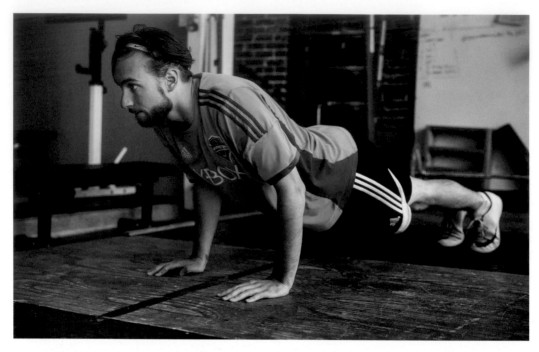

I was relieved that we didn't have to do weights for four rounds straight, even though I chose light hand weights. The 20-second bursts sound simple enough, but I'll tell you right now that the 10-second rests are not restful in the least. While the training calls for going as hard as possible during the intervals, I paced myself. With the music and constant cardio, the class felt hyper and more nonstop than Tabata alone feels. With fist pumps, feet scissoring, and jumping on and off the stepper, it was an amped-up aerobics class.

I loved some exercises with the stretchy bands, looping a band around my ankles and lifting one out side to side to work our outer adductors. Vaulting over the stepper also was fun, and a nice break from constant weight work.

My quads and hamstrings felt the intensity of squats with hand weights, and my triceps wished the teachers hadn't singled them out. I was right about the felt cloth pieces—we put the felt under our feet, put our hands on the stepper to get into a plank, and slid our feet in and out to work our cores.

My inner complainer had plenty of evidence that the class was difficult. Still, I was more entertained than if I had done Tabata alone at home. The high-energy music and folks who bounced or jogged during the 10-second rests pushed me to keep going. The best part of Tabata is it tricks you with the 20-second intervals; it's mentally easier to go hard for such a short stint.

By the end of class, I felt fully depleted, which is sometimes exactly what I want.

Tabata is an effective, short workout, and it's easy to do without added weights. It's useful if you have a short attention span or if you have kids and need to get in a workout at home that doesn't take the two hours it might take to get to and from a gym. It's also easy to squeeze in when traveling, when time truly can be limited and you want to get in strengthening as well as a cardiovascular challenge. While it may sound like a simple workout, it is intense, even when you're in good shape.

And sometimes, being efficient is the highest priority. Those times, Tabata it is.

GET STARTED WITH TABATA

Choose two bodyweight exercises (see sidebar) and do an eight-minute Tabata workout, timing yourself for 20 seconds on and 10 seconds off. Do this once a week until you're ready to move to the Level Up goal.

BEFORE YOU GO

Equipment: Sneakers, comfortable clothes.
Cost: Drop-in fees for Tabata classes vary from studio to studio but average around $10 to $25 per class.

CHALLENGE YOURSELF

Once you've built up some endurance and strength doing a couple of exercises at a time, mix up the exercises to challenge yourself. See if you can meet these goals:

Level Up: Do a full round of Tabata with five bodyweight exercises once a week.

QUICK TIPS

- If you're still new to moving regularly, make sure you have a strong baseline of fitness before diving into a full Tabata workout. Start with one or two exercises and see how it feels to work this intensely before doing a complete workout on your own. It's also smart to take a class where a trainer can keep an eye on you as you learn the workout.
- For a Tabata workout at home, look online for free Tabata timers to make it easy to stay true to 20 seconds on, 10 seconds off.
- You can use the Tabata protocol for any kind of exercise, like running intervals or riding an indoor bike. Whatever the exercise, the protocol raises your heart rate immediately, and your body will have to work hard to keep up with the intensity.

Reach Goal: Do Tabata twice a week, and change up the bodyweight exercises. Check online for a wealth of ideas for how to work out using your own body's weight, including lunges, pull-ups, side plank holds, burpees, and jumping squats. Mix Tabata with straight cardio by running intervals or using a rower or an indoor bike.

Adventure Goal: Add weights to challenge yourself even more. Use small hand weights for leg workouts or hold a kettlebell for squats.

DISCOVERY: *Tabata*

	1ST	2ND	3RD
DATE			
DURATION			
RATING (1 TO 5 STARS)	★ ★ ★ ★ ★	★ ★ ★ ★ ★	★ ★ ★ ★ ★

Do you typically think working out takes too much time? What did you find out about the time it takes to do a Tabata workout?

What did you learn about ways to get stronger every day through a Tabata workout?

Did you find the short bursts of effort easier to stick with or more challenging?

Month **11**

Snowshoeing

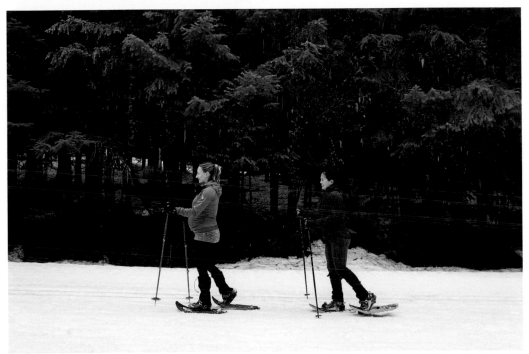

When I am out in snow, when the noise of the world and chatter of my mind are muffled by a deep white blanket, I soften. I no longer mind the cold. I breathe more deeply. Layer in the light of a moon, its bright outline enhanced by the dark sky, and the romantic in me falls hard. So when I saw that a local outdoor store offered a moonlight snowshoe, I knew I had to go.

Of all the snow sports, snowshoeing is the most beginner friendly. It is also low impact

and can be quite aerobic if you're on a steeper trail; it offers many of the benefits of walking or hiking. Because snowshoeing may take you into the backcountry, it's also important to be aware of and prepared for potential avalanche danger (see sidebar).

The one element that can stop me from heading out to move during the colder months is gear. Winter sports, in particular, require a lot of gear, from snowshoes and poles to the layering and bundling required to be outside for several hours. This is in addition to the driving time needed to get to the mountains.

The best thing about going with my local outfitter was that they drove us to the trailhead. Plus, they showed up with a van full of the latest snowshoes, poles, and gaiters. And our group had leaders who kept an eye on weather and avalanche conditions to make sure we stayed safe—and as a bonus, they stopped at a local bakery for a treat.

We arrived at the trailhead after dark and got a quick talk on staying warm and safe while snowshoeing. We had received an email detailing what to wear and how to layer in winter, and the leaders reviewed why: wear a first layer like wool or a synthetic that wicks sweat, add another two warm layers to keep heat in, and then put on a waterproof shell to stay dry from falling snow or other moisture.

I tracked everything leaders Kevin and David said until they told us not to sweat. I hadn't heard of this insanity. How do you not sweat when snowshoeing uphill? Vent, they said. Take off a layer when you get warm. That way, your body cools, and you don't sweat. Sweat will make you cold.

AVALANCHE SAFETY

Avalanche education is for everyone, not just people who go into the backcountry. Many people have the misperception that snowshoeing is less risky than backcountry skiing, but you're still in the same mountain terrain as skiers and snowmobilers. It's important to understand when you're in avalanche territory and at risk.

Three things are needed to launch snow down a slope: terrain, triggers, and unstable snow.

Humans are a trigger, adding stress to snow. Snowpack can become unstable from wind, a really fast snowfall (12 inches or more in 24 hours elevates risk), and rain or quick temperature changes. Snowpack needs time to adjust before it's considered stable again, according to the Northwest Avalanche Center.

Check local avalanche center websites, which monitor snowpack and conditions. Terrain matters. Avalanches happen on 30- to 45-degree slopes. Flatter slopes aren't steep enough for snow to slide. If they're steeper than 45 degrees, the snow slides constantly. In between, 30 to 45 degrees is steep enough to hold snow *and* for it to slide.

You can increase safety by traveling with a group that communicates well. Does everyone have the same goals? Does everyone have avalanche training and equipment, including an avalanche beacon and a shovel? Is everyone doing research on snow conditions and terrain? Will everyone decide as a group their risk tolerance?

If you devote yourself to a backcountry sport, experts advise taking a more in-depth avalanche course where you learn to "read" slopes and terrain.

Always carry a probe, an avalanche beacon, and a shovel, and know how to use them. If you're buried four or five feet under the snow, your group will have to shovel between one ton and one and half tons of snow to get to you. The message: whatever you do, take precautions and do your best not to get caught in an avalanche.

Not sweating seemed an impossible task, especially on a snowshoe trip I expected to be vigorous. But then they also reminded us not to get cold. They told us to warm up and get blood out to our fingers and toes by jumping around if we did get cold. Maintaining the right body temperature sounded complicated, but I decided to figure it out along the way.

After a quick rundown on gear, we put on our snowshoes and snapped on gaiters to cover our ankles and keep the snow out of our boots. I've had a pair of snowshoes collecting dust in my closet, and I was happy to put them to use.

Snowshoes have teeth that grip when you are on ice or snow and are wide to keep you from sinking into soft snow. They are so wide that you may feel slightly bow-legged walking to accommodate the large, awkward objects strapped to your feet. You might trip once or twice; I did in the parking lot. But once you get used to walking slightly wider than normal, it's straightforward.

We spread out and started walking, with one leader in front and one leader bringing up the rear. We tackled a fairly steep climb right away. The biggest challenge in a group outing is pace, and how fast you move together as a group depends on everyone's level of skill and conditioning. Kevin, who led us up, kept the pace on the slower side to make sure the group stuck together. I like to go fast on trails and wanted to move more quickly. When I got on the heels of the person in front of me a couple of times, I reminded myself I was on the outing to enjoy myself, not to win any speed records.

After a while, I stopped wishing we would go faster and I started looking around instead.

I loved the crisp, piney scent of the dark woods surrounding the trail and the feel of cold, snowy air in my nose and lungs. Our leaders had strung battery-powered holiday lights on their backpacks, both festive and easy to spot. Our headlights bounced through the dark woods, the tree branches overhead heavy with snow. It was beautiful and quiet as our snowshoes squeaked over the thick snow.

We crossed a couple creeks, and again our leaders offered helpful advice, telling us exactly where to step on snow bridges. I could hear water moving underneath us and liked having someone else making sure I made it across without getting wet.

At our pace, the snowshoe was not strenuous, though there was plenty of uphill—more than 1,000 feet of elevation gain over 1.5 miles—for my heart rate to pick up and to stay warm. Snowshoes spread out the impact on your body, both on the uphill and downhill, so even with the incline, it felt easy on my joints. I almost started to sweat and remembered to pull off a layer.

It was cloudy that night, but once we made it to the lake, we could make out the full moon through the dark clouds. We stood on the edge of the frozen lake, eating sandwiches we had packed and drinking celebratory fizzy apple juice the leaders had hauled up.

Our pace was faster on the way down. Everyone seemed eager to get back to the bus for the long drive back.

Snowshoeing at night is dreamy. The short trip took longer than it would have on my own, but I'm not sure I would do it at night even with one or two other people. With a group of 10, it felt fun and adventurous, without any of the worry I might otherwise have in the dark. I loved having guides experienced with avalanche safety. I especially loved having a bus and guides who drove us there and back.

If you're looking to try out snowshoeing, go for the snow, for the adventure, and if you time it right, for the full moon.

GET STARTED SNOWSHOEING

Rent snowshoes, gaiters, and poles, and head out to a flat trail to get used to walking on snowshoes.

QUICK TIPS

- Gaiters are essential for keeping the snow out of your boots and staying dry. Purchase a pair or rent them before you head out.
- Carry plenty of food and water. You'll be working hard, and your body needs fuel and hydration.
- Make sure you go with a group and that everyone is prepared with equipment, layers, water, food, and other essentials. Don't snowshoe alone.
- Always check the weather and trail conditions before you go.

BEFORE YOU GO

Equipment: Snowshoes, poles, waterproof boots, gaiters, warm layers (no cotton).
Cost: Renting snowshoes can cost anywhere from $15 to $35. Check your local trail organizations to see if you need a day pass for parking or to pay for a groomed trail, which can start around $10 per day.

CHALLENGE YOURSELF

When snowshoeing, you can increase intensity through both elevation gain and the length of the trail. Once you're used to walking with snowshoes on flat terrain, work up to these goals:

Level Up: Look for a local outdoor group or retailer that hosts beginner snowshoe treks. Sign up for one for the experience and the guidance.

Reach Goal: Take an avalanche awareness course so you know the signs and understand how to keep yourself safe. Then go out on more challenging trails with steeper elevation gain.

Adventure Goal: Take a backcountry snowshoe course and learn the skills required to go off trails and out on your own.

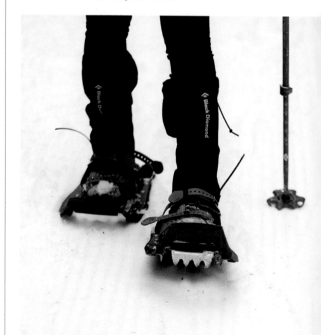

DISCOVERY: *Snowshoeing*

	1ST	2ND	3RD
DATE			
DURATION			
RATING (1 TO 5 STARS)	★ ★ ★ ★ ★	★ ★ ★ ★ ★	★ ★ ★ ★ ★

What did you appreciate about being outside in the cold and snow and moving through the woods on snowshoes?

If you are a person who already enjoys outdoor snow sports, snowshoeing provides an opportunity to slow down. What was different about snowshoeing versus a faster-paced sport like skiing?

Were you able to snowshoe without sweating? What did you discover about the kind of effort involved in snowshoeing?

Were you surprised by any element of the experience, from how it felt to being prepared for the weather or what you enjoyed or disliked? Why?

Tai Chi

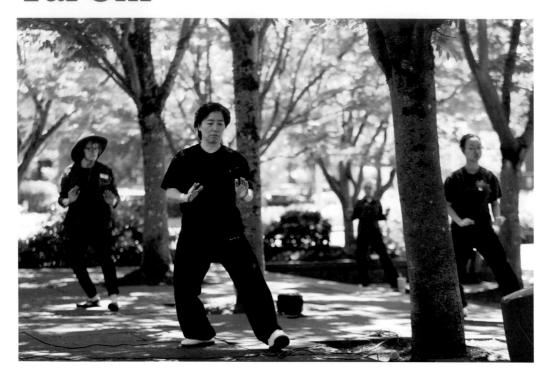

The class moved with precision, most of the students flowing with intention and focus through the forms. I, on the other hand, looked around wondering what it meant to "grasp the sparrow's tail."

I was at a local senior center to take tai chi chuan (or taiji quan), a Chinese martial art that includes breathwork and martial arts movements that challenge balance and control. Tai chi is one of the internal martial arts and falls under the umbrella of qigong.

Tai chi movement is slow and fluid, with a focus on shifting weight from foot to foot and rotating the body in various directions, all of which help retain balance and function, particularly useful for older folks. It also requires you to concentrate on breathing and slowing down movement.

Qigong is the father martial art to tai chi. *Qi* is translated from Chinese as "vital energy." If you're interested in knowing more about the roots of tai chi, look for a qigong class.

Tai chi tends to be more vigorous and active, whereas qigong includes seated meditation plus a moving practice. Some teachers consider qigong so important that they require tai chi students to study it.

Researchers have found that seniors who practiced tai chi twice a week for 12 weeks had improved gait, balance, and overall function. One study showed that seniors who took tai chi had 49 percent fewer falls.

At the senior center, the regulars attended class twice a week with their teacher, Susan, who specializes in the yang style of tai chi. Many students have practiced with her for years, and it showed in their familiarity with the movements. The yang style has 24 forms, or sections—with several movements per form—and it takes roughly a year to learn with weekly practice, according to Master Yijiao Hong of the Chinese Wushu and Taichi Academy in Seattle.

Susan took the senior center class through warm-ups, then moved right into that week's form. I tried to stay on pace, craning my head to see how to "part the wild horse's mane."

I was relieved when we paused to drill a few movements. We focused first on our hips.

Susan told us to relax and loosen our hips and to notice how the movement felt in our knees and ankles. I felt my weight sink toward my feet. She said to let our wrists and elbows get heavy, and my arms and shoulders heard the signal, relaxing more toward the ground. We practiced shifting our weight from one foot to the other and did some footwork, moving 70 percent of our weight to one side, for example. Keep your centerline of gravity over one foot at a time, Susan instructed.

The slow movements helped me feel how to stay balanced on one foot, particularly during a move when we kicked one foot out. All of the students managed the kick with aplomb.

We also practiced moving our hands through different positions, and Susan quizzed the students on their names, including earth, water, fire, metal.

Next, Susan walked us through "needle at the bottom of the sea." We started with our weight on one foot, moved forward with one arm to block an invisible opponent's attack, shifted our weight again to the other foot, and let our hands relax—or at least that's what I retained from the various cues flooding my ears.

TAI CHI STYLES

There are many styles of tai chi practiced and taught in the United States; the following are the three most popular ones. The styles are more similar than they are different, all focusing on building your qi energy using slow, flowing movements.

YANG: The most widely practiced style, yang tai chi is relatively simple and easy to learn with big, open movements that are centered, calm, and steady.

WU: This style of tai chi focuses on smaller, compact movement to build and retain energy.

CHEN: This is the oldest form, alternating bursts of dynamic movement with slower motions; it is more physical than other styles of tai chi.

I was impressed watching some of the older students balance on one foot for extended periods of time, not an easy skill regardless of age. Relaxing my ribs to twist my torso side to side was more difficult than it sounded. Susan pointed out how hips, ankles, and feet move for balance, and she instructed us to use our upper bodies for balance and twists. The slow focus moves the body into a parasympathetic recovery-and-repair mode, she said.

After the drills, we went through the entire 20-movement form again, just one piece of the full set of 24 forms. I felt more grounded after the drills and focused on centering my weight rather than worrying too much about my hand shape. I started to get the feel for a few movements, like holding an energy ball between my hands and boxing imaginary ears.

I was the youngest one attending class that day, but age had no bearing on ability, at least not in this class. The regulars had an ease and elegance rooted in years of practice, as I did my best to mimic everyone else and remember what came next.

A 74-year-old gentleman in the class, Ken, had been doing tai chi for seven years. He'd started taking class to maintain balance, with the goal to "stay upright as long as I can." The biomechanics of the body interested him, and he liked learning more about how the body works and how people move. He learned enough to do some of the forms on his own, he said. While tai chi is often geared toward seniors, it is an art form you can take on at any age.

I returned to tai chi a few years later in an introductory class with Master Hong. Some movements felt familiar as she took us through breathing exercises and paying

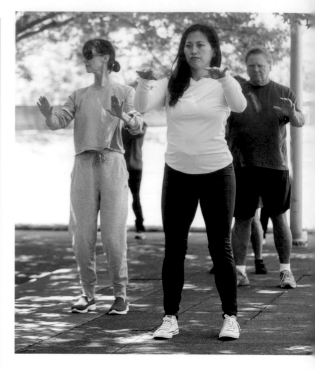

attention to the energy and movement of our arms, slowly lifting them forward until they were parallel with our shoulders and then slowly settling them back down beside our hips. She showed us how to use our arms to pull an imaginary opponent toward us in a defensive move.

The nuances of the movements make a difference, like bringing your chin to a level that is "elegant, not arrogant," Master Hong said. I turned my attention to feeling the pull of gravity in my hands. As with the first time I took tai chi, the focus on relaxing my elbows, hands, and shoulders helped me home in on my body and calmed my mind.

Next, Master Hong showed us the three major stances, starting in the bow-and-arrow stance (akin to a short warrior 1 in yoga) and how to shift weight to the empty stance (where all the weight moves to your back foot) and then switch to the T-stance (where weight transfers again to one foot, the other one light on the ground). From there, we moved back to bow and arrow.

It all started to click. I could see the rhythm and reason for the foot patterns as we moved through a full form.

At the close of class, Master Hong and some students demonstrated the 24 forms. Tai chi is more than balance and grace; there was incredible artistry to their movement and their mental focus. I watched as they went through deep, controlled lunges, did slow kicks, and moved their hands into graceful positions.

Their concentration through the five or so minutes it took to get through all the forms was visible on their faces, their eyes focused and their breath steady. I could see why it takes a full year to learn the complex movements that make up all 24.

Tai chi trains muscles to be flexible and strong, but you also build an overall sense of balance and serenity. "When mind and body calm, breath is longer," said Master Hong. "It's the breathing we want for longevity."

I appreciated the equanimity I felt at the end of class, something I don't always build into my day. The slow movement also helped me notice my balance and challenged it at the same time. It's a practice that anyone can benefit from.

GET STARTED WITH TAI CHI

Take an intro class at a local studio or look for a beginner tai chi class at a community center.

QUICK TIPS

- There are many styles of tai chi (see sidebar). If you have various options available, consider trying different styles before settling on one.
- Watch online videos that teach some of the essential movements, helpful for practicing between classes.

BEFORE YOU GO

Equipment: Comfortable clothes to move in and sneakers or other comfortable shoes.
Cost: The fee for a class depends on whether you go to a studio or a community center; the range is from $5 to $15, with community centers offering the most affordable options.

CHALLENGE YOURSELF

Learning the forms takes time. The challenge comes from adding new forms over time. After you've tried an intro class, do these:

Level Up: Take a tai chi class once a week for a month and build an understanding of the movements in a form.
Reach Goal: Take class twice a week and learn two forms this month. Practice at home to develop a greater understanding and knowledge of this ancient martial art.
Adventure Goal: Add in a qigong class to gain a deeper connection to energy and how it moves in your body.

DISCOVERY: *Tai Chi*

	1ST	2ND	3RD
DATE			
DURATION			
RATING (1 TO 5 STARS)	★ ★ ★ ★ ★	★ ★ ★ ★ ★	★ ★ ★ ★ ★

What was the most physically challenging part of your first tai chi class? Was it balance, or was it the pace?

Were you able to appreciate the pace of class, or did you struggle to stay engaged with a slower movement? Why?

How did you feel at the end of class after spending time focusing on breathing and slowing down the movements of your body? Did you notice a shift in energy from the start of class to the end?

What did you learn about your expectations of what exercise and movement are supposed to be like and how it compared to what you experienced in tai chi?

Month **12**

Skiing

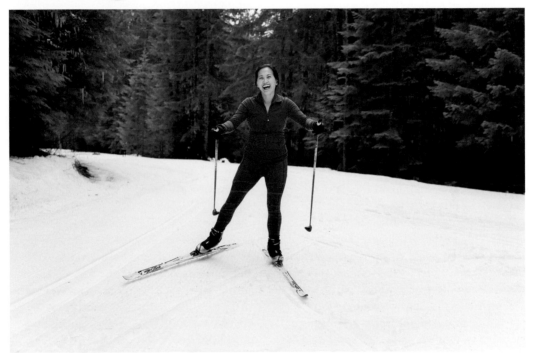

When I first learned to cross-country ski, I skipped classic technique and went straight to the speedier skate style, where instead of moving your feet along parallel tracks, you push off in a V-shape in a movement similar to ice skating, only with skis. I liked how fast I could go by skate skiing, pushing hard through my feet to gain momentum and speed.

I could especially see the difference when I was on the uphills, flying past classic skiers who were moving along parallel tracks groomed into the snow next to the smooth trail I was using for skate skiing. When I went skate skiing with friends who were on classics, I impatiently waited for them at the top of each hill, ready to fly downhill again.

Many years later, I decided I had been unfair in dismissing the classic skiing technique. It was time to give it a chance, so I headed to a local ski center, which had received a fluffy layer of snow ideal for a cross-country ski. Classic skiing is like a formal dance, the local snow sports manager told me. Take your time on refining technique, and practice getting all your weight on one foot at a time. Learning classic technique would help improve my skate skiing, he added. I nodded. Still, I felt my skate skier's impulse to race up hills bubbling up to the surface. I quelled it, telling myself I would have fun slowing it down.

First, I had to understand the equipment. Sharon, my instructor, explained the essential components of a classic ski. The base—unlike the smooth underside of a skate ski—has scales in the middle, which grip snow on slick uphills. The camber, or flex in the middle of the ski, gives you a loaded spring action to move forward. When you push off, press down into the middle of the ski, she explained.

We practiced the technique on a small, flat loop. Pretend you're a teenager sneaking into the house late at night, Sharon said. I did my best imitation of my 16-year-old self, creeping back home from a late-night party with friends. Suddenly, Sharon shouted, "Run!" I started jogging, going as fast as I could on my skis, and was soon breathless. This classic ski thing was not as easy as I thought.

After a few laps working on my teenage stealth moves, Sharon said I was thinking too much about my hands. She took away my poles. Wait, what? I need those for balance, I protested meekly.

I wobbled at first, unsteady without their help, as I tried to slink back into my parents' house. Now that I couldn't rely on the poles, my balance improved.

I graduated to going uphill. You need to angle your body roughly 90 degrees from the slope of the hill to take advantage of the ski, Sharon said. This did not seem like good advice.

Let your butt pull your weight down toward your feet, she said, instead of leaning forward, which is what I wanted to do. I soon found out that if you lean forward, you slide backward, which happened a few times. Fine, Sharon. I'll do it your way.

When a hill gets steep, sometimes you herringbone your way up, stepping your feet in a V-shape up the hill, a shape I knew from skate skiing. So when Sharon suggested we go uphill to some flatter terrain and offered me the option of taking a ski lift, I suggested we go the steep way and practice herringbone technique. I had no illusions at this point that this would be easy on my legs, but I thought more practice was better. I charged up the hill—at times tempted to skate up—but didn't regret my choice.

On the trail, Sharon watched me ski and told me how I could refine my technique. After you push off, your back heel lifts up and you glide forward. My back foot was not getting far enough forward past my front foot with each step, limiting my glide. I focused on relaxing my toes, bending my knees and punching my front foot a little farther forward with each push.

I also was stiff in my lower back. The more I softened, the easier it would be, Sharon said. She introduced a technique where I pushed with one foot and then double-poled forward. It was a little hard to get the rhythm down, but once you get it, you can go much faster. I concentrated and was able to pick up some speed.

Even with the technical work, at moments I remembered to look around. The scent of fresh pine wafted across the snowy trail, and a light

OR TRY . . . SNOWBOARDING

On snow, I am most comfortable when my feet are operating independently on two skis, not glued to one board.

Still, so many people love snowboarding that I decided to get over my reluctance, and my friend Katie and I headed up to a local ski resort to try out the sport. Once we slid our feet into our boots and made it outside, it was exhilarating to watch skiers and snowboarders flying down snowy runs. I loved the smell of cold snow and crisp mountain air.

In class, Katie and I were the elders among all the kids and teenagers. We started out learning to stay upright, and then how to use edges on a gentle slope. I found it disconcerting to have my body face one direction and my head another. We practiced carving slow turns, shifting weight between our toes and heels to control where we were headed, in theory.

I had heard I would spend most of my first time on my butt or knees. I had a few good falls but felt cheerful about my balance.

Our technique improved throughout the class. Once our lesson was done, we got on the chairlift for longer runs, though I was more terrified of falling off the lift.

Our first run was slow. Speed and balance don't go hand in hand. Falling involved hysterical giggles. Bit by bit, we got the hang of it. I struggled to carve into my heels, and it was scary to lean into my front foot and the downhill for speed, but I made it down with minimal wipeouts.

I emerged from the day tired and happy. It was less painful than I thought. Strap both feet to one board and see what you can learn about strength and balance.

snow fell on my shoulders. There was a deep hush around us from the new layer of snow, muting sound from other skiers.

The greatest benefit to classic skiing, beyond spending your lifetime refining technique, is you can go all day, Sharon said, a more difficult challenge with skate skis. After an hour of skate skiing, I was ready for a break. I liked the idea of skiing into the woods for a long day of adventure and exploration.

Both classic and skate technique rely on balance, all your weight on one foot at a time to get more glide and momentum. I was happy that classic technique, which is easy on the joints, was still a vigorous workout. I can see how this is a sport that lasts a lifetime—no need to say more.

Still, you may find the meditative aspect of cross-country skiing not quite enough. Or, you may simply prefer the thrill of the downhill and want the physical intensity required to do turns down a steep slope. So let's talk downhill skiing.

Skiing of any style, whether alpine or cross-country, is a mix of endurance and resistance training that requires balance to navigate slick conditions and core strength to keep yourself upright. Cross-country tends to be more aerobic, whereas alpine skiing requires bursts of strength, building leg strength through resistance to gravity as you shush down steep slopes.

I learned to alpine ski on a former landfill in Wisconsin. Those hills passed for elevation in the Midwest. My parents drove us from our home in Illinois to Wisconsin a couple of times on ski trips—there are old family photos of me decked out in a puffy coat, thick snow pants, and ski goggles. Not having honed my skills on steep, dramatic mountains as one childhood friend had in Colorado, when I arrived at college in New Hampshire, I knew I would have to start from the beginning.

I took intro skiing classes, piling onto a bus every weekend to head up to my college's ski hill. There, I learned the basics, starting with snowplowing on bunny hills and moving into turns in an inverted V-shape. I was embarrassed sometimes as brand-new friends whizzed down the slopes carving turns, and I watched from the chairlift as their hair flew out from under their helmets. But it motivated me; I was determined to get better at skiing.

Trails rated for cross-country and alpine use the same color system. You start with the greens for the beginner level and master your technique, then move on to blue trails—or if you have up-leveled your skill set, black—to add challenge. I disliked being a beginner, but the first time we got on the chairlift and I faced my first blue hill, I was happy I had a teacher guiding me.

Our teacher coached us down the steeper portions, helping us with turns and how to transfer our weight forward. Unlike cross-country skiing, my teacher wanted me to lean into the downhill slope, which was terrifying. What if I don't want to go faster?

But that's not how it works when your aim is to get down a steep hill. So, week after week, I worked on my turns, learning to plant my pole and turn around it, wending my way downhill. Control was often dicey, especially on the icy New England slopes. But I slowly progressed, spending days I didn't have classes on the bus and slopes with my friend Alice, who was a beginner snowboarder, to get some runs in.

The steeper the hills got, the deeper the burn in my thighs on the way down, and the bigger the rush. Sometimes, as I crouched into my ski stance, leaning forward into the rush of the downhill, I wondered how long my legs could last in that position.

I never got addicted to the rush, though I did love the feeling of a snowy wind brushing my face and the sharpness of cold air in my lungs. I practically hooted when I nailed a turn rather than skidding through it. I started to relax, confident that I could at least navigate my way down a mountain.

After college, cross-country skiing replaced alpine skiing for me. But I can vouch that each will take you into the wilderness, into fresh air, and into challenge. If you're curious, consider the challenge of trying both and seeing which is a better fit. You can't go wrong.

GET STARTED SKIING

Look for introductory classes at a ski resort, Nordic center, or with local outdoor club to become familiar with the equipment and learn how to move around with long skis on your feet. If you haven't done it before, it's awkward!

BEFORE YOU GO

Equipment: For both cross-country and alpine skiing, you'll need boots, skis, poles, plus a hat, gloves, and warm socks. For cross-country, you'll want warm, comfortable, waterproof clothes in layers that you can easily adjust as you warm up and cool down. For alpine skiing, you'll need a helmet and goggles; waterproof, insulated ski pants and coat will keep you warm on chilly rides on the chair lift. **Cost:** For cross-country, equipment rentals for boots, skis, and poles average $35 to $45. Some resorts offer a package that includes a trail pass and rentals. Groomed trails managed independently of resorts may require a pass to cover the cost of grooming, roughly $10 to $20 depending on the location. For alpine, the costs are higher, with equipment rentals averaging around $50 and day passes ranging $60 to $120. Look for package deals that include rentals and lessons for the day.

CHALLENGE YOURSELF

Once you've gotten comfortable on your skis, challenge yourself with harder trails or additional classes.

Level Up: Once you can comfortably cruise green trails on your own, tackle some blue trails. **Reach Goal:** Depending on how much time you have, progress to the next class level. If you're spending a weekend or a few days at a snowy location, look for ways to move up to intermediate classes and then practice afterward. If you've been taking classic ski lessons, try a skate skiing class.
Adventure Goal: For cross-country, go out for a full day of skiing. Map out your trails and make sure you understand avalanche awareness (see sidebar in "Snowshoeing") if you're on classic skis and going into the backcountry. Be sure to bring a good map and GPS device or app, and let someone know where you'll be. For alpine skiers, take on some new, more difficult terrain and challenge yourself to fly a little faster.

QUICK TIPS

- Be aware that ski sports require a significant investment, from the cost of equipment to having warm, waterproof clothing plus goggles for alpine skiers and snowboarders. Until you're committed to either sport beyond a couple of attempts, just rent equipment.
- The beauty of cross-country skiing is that the technology doesn't change much. Once you invest in a set of skis, bindings, boots, and poles, you're set. Alpine ski technology moves at a fast clip. If you invest in a full set of boots, bindings, skis, and poles, within a couple of years, you may want to upgrade as better skis come out. All alpine ski areas rent skis and typically carry the latest technology to try out. Ski swaps and shopping at the end of the season are ways to find deals on equipment.
- Though you can rent a pair of skis and go out on your own with no instruction, I don't recommend this route; it's the pathway to frustration, a lot of wipeouts, and potentially an early end to your nascent skiing career. If you've never skied before, take a class and learn the basics right the first time.

DISCOVERY: *Skiing*

	1ST	2ND	3RD
DATE			
DURATION			
RATING (1 TO 5 STARS)	★ ★ ★ ★ ★	★ ★ ★ ★ ★	★ ★ ★ ★ ★

Are you more inclined toward a meditative pace with cross-country skiing or the rush of alpine skiing? Why?

What did you discover about your balance in your first ski class?

If this is your first time doing a snow sport, what was your favorite aspect of being outside in the winter? What did you find challenging?

What would motivate you to go skiing again? Why?

Pilates

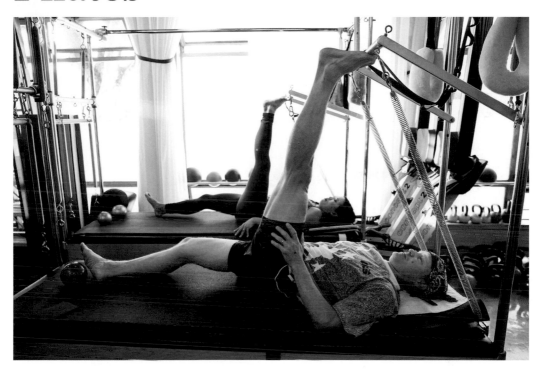

I had not experienced Pilates like this before. A disco ball hung overhead. The music was loud. I was dripping sweat, and I'm pretty sure I grunted.

Pilates and I have a tumultuous history. I know Pilates has benefits for strengthening weak muscles that escape my notice. But I struggle to stay interested in all the muscles I'm required to engage for good form. As much as I love anatomy, form, and strength, Pilates and I haven't clicked.

I'm always on the hunt for a Pilates approach that I might come to enjoy, so when a trainer recommended an interval class, describing it as "CrossFit mixed with Pilates," and a real butt kicker, I perked up. Those are fighting words to me.

A Pilates class is a series of exercises with specific form and alignment designed to build strength and increase mobility and is known for targeting your core. Studies show that Pilates can not only improve balance and

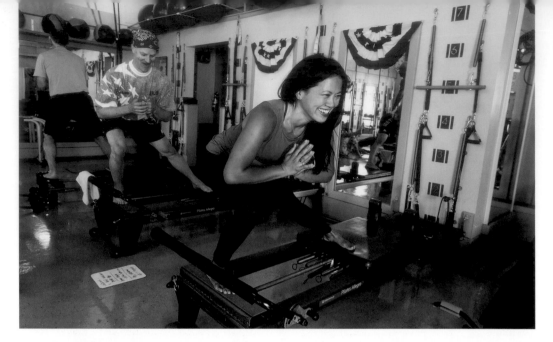

strength but can also help with lower back pain. Some research has shown it also helps with flexibility, trunk stability, and injury prevention.

While Pilates uses several types of machines that help isolate different muscle groups, there are also mat classes that rely on Pilates techniques without the machines. The form for Pilates is specific, and an experienced teacher will make a difference in how much you get out of a class.

I was originally interested in the AMRAP Pilates class, which takes its name from a CrossFit term "as many rounds as possible," but timing worked out for the interval class. Based on what I know now, I'm glad I didn't make it to the AMRAP class.

Owner Dana has been teaching Pilates for years and weaves in his own experience from cross-functional fitness. He sets up stations at various machines with four rounds (or more) of each exercise for 30 seconds on, then a buzzer for a brief interval of rest, before you move to the next station and a new exercise. You go through all the machines, from the classic Pilates Reformer with straps, springs, and sliding platforms to the Wunda Chair (see sidebar), essentially a box with a moving step. The class also mixes in some exercises on a mat.

I buddied up with teacher Verna, who helped me with machines and technique. After a warm-up round with a lot of core under Dana's watchful eye, we started the first full round with goblet squats (deep squats holding a kettlebell) for 30 seconds on, 10 seconds off. I can do weighted squats for four rounds, no problem, I thought. I felt confident, probably more than was justified.

We moved on to weighted oblique work, rolling onto one side, holding a medicine ball, and lifting for several reps. After that, we did a round of push-ups. I eyed the upcoming exercises and modified my push-ups with knees down.

With Pilates, core is a constant theme. During our core work, Dana prompted me to contract my front ribs in toward each other instead of puffing them out, a key part of a strong core that requires constant vigilance. I was also grateful when he came by and unhooked a spring or two on a Pilates Reformer to make my workout easier. When one station called for simple side stretches, I happily sighed into the stretch.

By the time I got to ticktocks (moving a weightlifting bar side to side in a side lunge), my heart rate was elevated and my muscles ached. I hoped the next full series of exercises would be easier. I should have known better.

Our first station started with ring rows, followed by jumping lunges. You can mix them with jumping squats, Verna offered helpfully, as I gasped during the 30-second interval. I no longer wanted to hold planks with TRX straps, nor did I want to hang by my elbows from a bar and pull my knees to my chest. Then I saw the incline sit-ups—

I may have groaned as Dana came over to instruct me to roll up and down as smoothly as possible.

The last few exercises included more core work sliding my feet back and forth on a blanket and a deep lunge exercise with one foot on an unstable surface to challenge stability in the glutes, ankle, and knee joints. When the ending buzzer rang, I already felt the muscular pangs that signaled pending soreness the next day.

But this Pilates playland changed my previous ho-hum attitude. We moved so fast from machine to machine that I was never bored. I liked the focus on technique and form; there was no encouragement to go faster than I was able. It was a Pilates class I could get down with.

PILATES, EXPLAINED

The class names at Pilates studios are typically based on the style of machines used in class. Here is a basic outline of class styles you may encounter.

MAT PILATES: The simplest version of Pilates, this class focuses on doing core strengthening exercises on the floor that target on your hips, back, abdominals, and glutes. Don't be deceived by the lack of equipment; you'll find these classes challenging.

REFORMER PILATES: This class incorporates the Reformer, a machine that uses sliding platforms and springs to increase or decrease resistance on exercises during class. Reformer exercises incorporate strength for your full body, with pushing and pulling for your upper body, and stability and strength for your lower body. Studios generally require an introduction to the machine before you can take a full Reformer class, and these classes are limited in size.

CIRCUIT PILATES: A circuit class will incorporate the Reformer and also will include other Pilates machines, such as the Wunda Chair, a stool-size machine with a platform that raises and lowers to build upper body and core strength. You also might see a Trapeze table, a platform with four attached poles designed to strengthen and open your hips and your spine. You also could see a Tower, which also uses sliding platforms and springs for additional strength and challenge.

I credit it with giving me the courage to return to a regular Pilates class.

The Power Reformer Lite class at a local fitness studio had potential for a non-Pilates convert. Teacher Marlys described it as a slow burn designed to fatigue your muscles while still incorporating Pilates form on a Reformer to intensify whatever exercises you're doing.

I could have guessed class would start with core, although I would rather do it at the beginning than the end. Marlys started us in a plank position on our elbows and placed our knees on a sliding platform that we moved back and forth to warm up our core. We added in balance by setting up on hands and knees, a strap looped around one foot. I extended my right leg straight back and moved it at a 45-degree angle to the right, hovering over the floor, before pulling it back in. My glutes and hips felt the effort.

The approach for every exercise was the same—move slowly and controlled for several counts. For the last eight counts, hold a position for added strength.

Slow burn, indeed.

We switched the strap to one hand and pulled it diagonally across our bodies, still on hands and knees, so we were sliding up and down the main frame of the Reformer. We lifted one leg for a hold to add in a balance challenge while still sliding up and down; I wobbled as I slid forward and back using the strap.

Next, we moved on to lunges, with one leg up on a moving platform on the Reformer and the other propped on the frame of the machine. We leaned forward holding hand weights, which adds core. I had to keep focus on my balance and my legs while sliding one

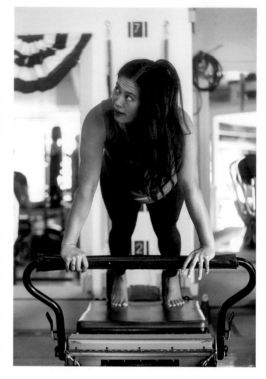

leg back and forth in deep lunges, and my glutes and legs burned even more.

By mid-class, my legs quaked as I slid one foot out on a platform. I was moving my foot in and out to work my inner thighs while simultaneously doing biceps curls with light weights. My body wanted out of all of these complicated movements and to stop shaking. I didn't know such excruciating physical sensation was possible. My inner thighs trembled, and I made sure I didn't slide my foot out so far that I would go into a split so deep I might never recover. My arms struggled to keep up with the curls and sometimes stopped moving as I gritted my teeth and tried not to lose control of my legs. During the final hold, legs in a split, knees bent, I breathed and hoped my leg on the sliding platform didn't give out. Then it was time to repeat the torture with the other leg.

We followed up with a glute exercise, and my fatigued lower body had to give in and take the occasional break. During class, I hadn't seen regulars taking breaks, so I tried not to. Later, Marlys assured me everyone takes a break at some point during the hour-long class.

We closed out class with a final plank hold, which, after the leg work, felt benign.

Despite some grumpiness mid-class, I liked the Power Reformer Lite class, which was much closer to a classic Pilates class but technically still less intense than a regular Reformer class. The exercises were so tough that my mind was engaged the whole time. The pacing also felt right, with a focus on form while moving through various exercises.

The great beauty of Pilates is the number of styles available. If the first class you take doesn't appeal to you, try another style. No matter what style you choose, your core will appreciate the challenge.

GET STARTED WITH PILATES

Take an introductory Reformer class or a mat class, which will get you plenty of core challenge without the complication of the machines.

BEFORE YOU GO

Equipment: Comfortable, stretchy clothes. Pilates is typically done barefoot or with socks with grips on the bottoms.
Cost: Drop-in classes vary from studio to studio, from $12 to $35.

QUICK TIPS

- There are many types of Pilates machines. Most studios offer an introductory class to teach you how to use the machines before you graduate into regular classes. I recommend taking one.
- Check out which types of Pilates classes are available in your area. There's a huge variety of styles out there (see sidebar); look for an approach that best suits you.

CHALLENGE YOURSELF

Once you've learned the basic form and how to use the machines, try these upgrades and you'll soon learn why Pilates is known for building strength, whether you stay with mat classes or move to Pilates machines.

Level Up: Go to class once or twice a week. If you haven't done Pilates before, you might be sore from just one class a week. If you're ready to ramp it up, go to two classes and see how strong you get.
Reach Goal: Take three classes a week and challenge yourself on new levels of strength.
Adventure Goal: See if there are other types of Pilates classes available, such as interval Pilates or heated Pilates, and expand your Pilates repertoire.

DISCOVERY: *Pilates*

	1ST	2ND	3RD
DATE			
DURATION			
RATING (1 TO 5 STARS)	★ ★ ★ ★ ★	★ ★ ★ ★ ★	★ ★ ★ ★ ★

What were your preconceptions about Pilates before going for the first time? What was it like in reality once you took the class?

I always find areas of weakness in my body during a Pilates class. What did you learn about your strength and where you can build more strength?

What did you appreciate about Pilates? Did you find anything challenging about the class? If, like me, you struggled with Pilates, what did you see about the advantage to this style of physical challenge?

Were you able to have fun during class? Why or why not?

RECOVERY: *Myofascial Release*

I use Yoga Tune Up Therapy Balls at home to roll out my feet. The squishy balls return to form even after you put your full weight on them. I love releasing tension in my arches or balls of my feet after a hike, when my feet are sore from miles on an uneven trail embedded with rocks and roots.

I also know the colorful rubber balls have more uses than for rolling out feet. I wanted to learn how to use them for myofascial release, a technique that releases tension in your connective tissue, or fascia. There are various ways to release tightness, from massage to self-myofascial release using tools like Therapy Balls.

I found a Yoga Tune Up class, led by Betsy, a Tune Up–certified instructor who teaches a combination of yoga and self-myofascial release. When I arrived at the class, Betsy told us we'd be using a pair of two-and-a-half-inch therapy balls, like the ones I owned, and a pair of three-and-a-half-inch alpha balls, which are larger and firmer than mine. She also asked what we wanted to work on—people mentioned hips, lower back, and shoulders. Another woman and I asked for feet.

To begin, Betsy had us lie down on our backs. The small therapy balls come with a little bag, and we each placed two small therapy balls in their enclosed bag on top of a yoga block and laid on it, just under the base of our skulls. This position moves your body into the parasympathetic state, slowing down your heart rate. It relaxes your muscles so the connective tissue is more receptive to rolling, Betsy explained.

I loved lying back on the balls. My breathing slowed, and I could feel my neck soften.

Next, we placed the balls, still in their bag, underneath our backs just inside one shoulder blade. I felt the balls push into tight tissue. Betsy had us inhale and exhale and slowly move one arm out onto the floor and then back across our chests.

I reveled in the shoulder opening and wondered why I'd never thought to use two balls at once, especially in this perpetually tight area of my body. We switched to the other shoulder blade, and I felt like I could do this movement forever.

But there was more to do. We took the balls out of the bag, placed them under the trapezoid muscles in our upper backs, and pushed against our feet into a bridge. This works the area affected when I stare at my computer, and the sensation was of intense relief.

Next, we rolled both sizes of the balls in the muscles around our upper and mid-spines. It was intense in a glorious way. Betsy reminded us to relax our faces as we rolled.

I was excited when we focused on our feet. I've sat in toes pose many times before, tucking my toes under me and sitting up on top of my feet to stretch the soles. Betsy intensified the pose by having us wrap a yoga strap around our ankles, securing our ankles together before sitting up on our feet like I was used to. When we released from the stretch, I wondered if I could walk afterward.

But now it was time to stand. I stepped on a smaller ball, and Betsy taught us to pause on points of tension and squish the ball from side to side to release. She had us pick up the ball with our toes for strengthening, though my toes didn't cooperate. I made a mental note to work on that at home.

We moved to our bellies to roll out quads and hip flexors, using a larger therapy ball. If there was a battle for tension between my upper back and quads, my thighs would put up a good fight. I almost yelped from the intensity. If we had more time, Betsy said, we would use the small therapy balls, too. I made another note to do this at home.

We finished with glutes, sitting with one small ball placed right into the tissue on each side to dig into the complex muscles and layers of fascia in our hips. I loved bending my legs and moving my knees side to side to release tightness that, let's face it, may never go away.

After class, Betsy told us we might be sore, so drink plenty of water to flush out toxins released during our session.

I came away with new ideas for using my therapy balls and have since bought more sizes, too. Betsy said myofascial release can be a daily practice, and the more you do it, the less intense it feels. I have rolled using techniques from this class ever since, and I can't say it's less intense—not yet. I also know how much better it makes me feel, so I don't let the intensity stop me.

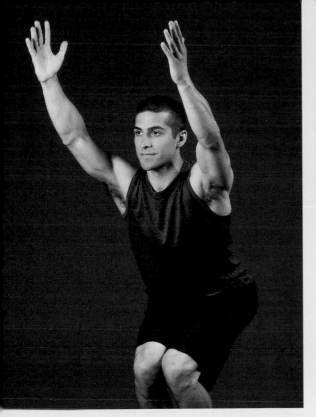
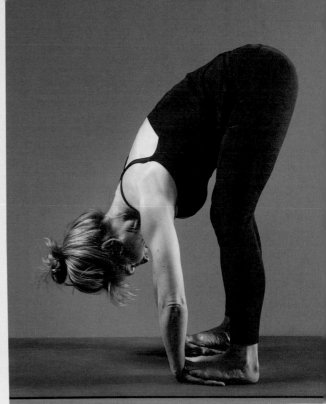

keep **it going** at **home**

Learning to move more outside of a yoga or fitness class has been one of my biggest shifts to staying healthy and fit. I love the challenge of a hard lifting session or sweaty yoga practice, and I also have learned that my body needs more movement than the one to two hours a day I spend at the gym or studio. Not only that, but I don't always have the two-plus hours required to get to a class, take it, and get home.

If you're inspired to take on new classes after reading this book, that is the goal. The reality is that you also may have a family or other commitments that make it difficult at times to do as much as you would like.

At those times, I follow the exercises and stretches below to give my body the movement it craves; in fact, I have built most of these movements into my day, every day. My body benefits as I tackle tight tissue, like in my feet, and it helps me mentally to know I am moving, especially if my schedule doesn't allow for a dedicated class.

Most of these are easy to add in at the end of the day as you're winding down. Do the exercises daily to make sure your body is getting a healthy dose of movement. Add in the stretches after dinner. Consider this an at-home improvement plan that you can follow no matter what month you're in or if you are traveling. Think of it as a way to keep yourself accountable to keep moving.

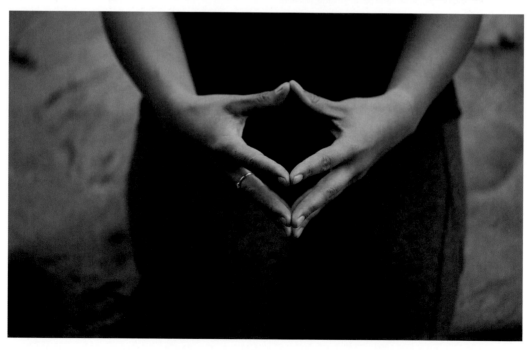

exercise at **home**

I am more motivated when I go to a gym or a class, but sometimes life gets busy and I might have only 20 minutes. If it's one of those days for you, take a 10-minute walk and follow with these exercises to move your body.

STRENGTHEN YOUR CORE

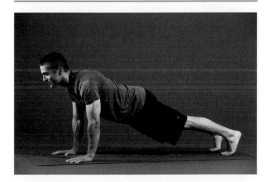

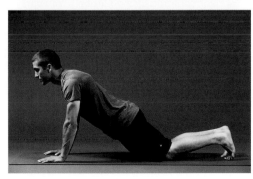

Your core, which extends from your pelvic floor to your neck, is the nexus of your body, and a strong core is the foundation for overall strength. It takes discipline to do core work at home, but I know you can do it. If you do only one core exercise every day, make it a plank.

To do a plank, get on your hands and knees on a mat or carpeted floor. Place your hands directly under your shoulders. Tuck your toes and straighten your legs behind you; lift your hips even with your shoulders to create a line from your feet to your shoulders. Press firmly into your hands, pushing into the floor until you feel your upper back muscles engage. Squeeze your thigh muscles, and pull your hands and feet toward each other for deeper core engagement. Lift your head so your neck is in line with the rest of your spine. Set a timer and hold for 30 seconds. Rest for 30 seconds, do it again.

Modification: Plank with your knees on the floor. Keep your hips in one line with your shoulders with your core engaged.

SIT ON THE FLOOR

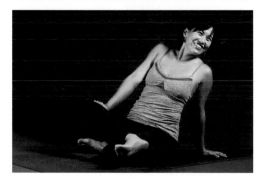

Moving off chairs and the couch onto the floor has created a monumental shift in how I hang out at home. When I'm on the couch, I can stay there for hours. The floor is more uncomfortable, which means I shift around and change the way I'm sitting rather than zoning out physically. Think of it as an antidote to all the sitting in chairs you've been doing during the day, whether it's at work or in the car. Add bolsters or pillows to the floor to make it more comfortable for stiff joints.

Sit on a cushion (or two) or a bolster, ankles crossed. Bring your hands to your glutes, feel around for the bones at the base of your pelvis and move your weight to the front side of your sitting bones. This action will help you get back the natural curve of your lumbar spine and sit up straighter. If crossing your ankles bothers your knees, extend one leg.

Bonus Movement: Lengthen your spine and contract your front ribs toward each other. Place one hand on the floor behind you (use a yoga block if you can't reach the floor) and turn your upper body toward that hand, adding a spinal twist.

STRETCH YOUR FEET

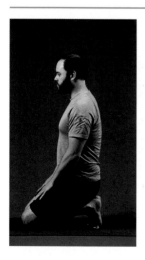

Moving your feet more is simple to do daily and has a major impact on your overall health. Your feet have one-quarter of the bones in your body and are most likely often encased in shoes that don't allow them to stretch or get stronger. Shifting your attention to your feet is one of the first steps I recommend to anyone interested in getting stronger and healthier. One easy step is to start wearing flat shoes. As you progress, look into shoes with a flexible sole and wide toe box to give your feet room to breathe.

To stretch your feet, do toes pose: Sit on your knees on a mat. Tuck your toes underneath you, making sure to tuck in your pinky toes, and then lift your chest over your hips until you feel the sensation. Breathe! This is an intense, deep stretch into the soles of your feet. Even if you can hold the stretch for only 10 seconds at first, it will be beneficial. Work up slowly until you can hold the stretch for 30 seconds.

IN THE MEANTIME:

- Take your shoes off and walk around barefoot.
- Stretch out your toes. Put a finger between every toe as spacers while you're watching your latest Netflix find.
- Step on a half-dome roller or place a folded-up towel under the balls of your feet to stretch your Achilles and calf. I work on this one frequently. Keep your weight centered over your heels. You can step one foot in front of the half-dome roller to intensify the stretch.
- Roll out your foot with a tennis ball or Yoga Tune Up Therapy Ball. Lightly roll the sole of your foot over the ball, and then find any spots that feel tight, step a little harder onto the ball, and massage that spot side to side.
- Want to bring in more movement at work? Take your shoes off and give your feet a break, or keep a roller ball under your desk to roll your feet out as you work.

SQUAT

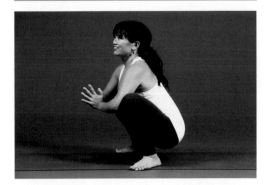

The squat is a bonanza for your ankles, hips, and pelvic floor, and it's a foundational movement for supporting a healthy spine and joints, but one that most of us don't do after childhood. Hours spent in a chair accumulate to limit this movement, so it can take time to work up to a deep squat, especially if you need to work on ankle or hip mobility.

Take your feet out wide and squat your hips down below your knees, if possible. Push your elbows into the insides of your knees, and hold the position. If you're hunching, as you press your elbows into your knees, see if you can lengthen your spine. You also can hold on to a chair or table leg to keep yourself in the squat.

If you have trouble squatting with your heels down or feet parallel, turn your toes out or widen your stance. You also can modify by folding a blanket or towel under your heels to ease the intensity and build up to a full squat, especially if you can't get your hips below your knees. Work up to a minute.

Challenge: Squat for 10 minutes a day. Don't do this all at once; find ways to squat for 30 seconds at a time throughout the day and keep track of your cumulative time so you get to 10 minutes.

WALK

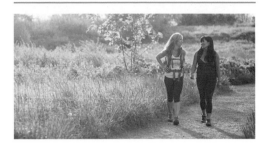

Walking is one of the most essential movements to do every day. No matter what else I do movement wise, I get in the four to four and a half miles needed to hit 10,000 steps. If I haven't reached this goal by the time I'm done with dinner, I'll take a short stroll around my neighborhood to get in my final steps.

Make your walks even more beneficial by turning them into tech-free time to give your ears and brain a break. Look out to the horizon to rest your eyes, too.

OTHER WAYS TO ADD WALKING INTO EVERY DAY:

- Park your car farther away from your destination, adding a five-minute walk every time you park.
- Set up walking meetings instead of sitting over coffee.
- Take transit instead of driving and add in more steps to and from work.
- Take a five-minute walk break at work every hour or in between meetings. It might feel like a lot of breaks, but remember that moving your body fuels your brain.
- Build a 15-minute walk into your lunch break.

stretch
at home

It takes time to increase mobility and blood flow in the areas of your body that get stuck from sitting all day. Incorporating the following stretches on a daily basis will help you over time.

You'll need minimal equipment: a mat, a block, and a bolster. If you don't have any of those, you can use the floor, blankets, and pillows you already have at home.

Even the most active people I know spend a large amount of time in a chair. It's the nature of our sedentary culture. You sit when driving, you sit for dinner, and you sit to watch television, not to mention one of the most common culprits—sitting at work.

What happens, exactly, when you sit so much?

HERE ARE A FEW OF THE IMPACTS:

- Weak glutes from lack of use
- Tight, contracted hamstrings from being in the same position
- Shortened hip flexors
- Disengaged, weakened core
- Rounded, tight shoulders
- Tight neck, from slumped shoulders and head protruding forward

SUPINE TWIST

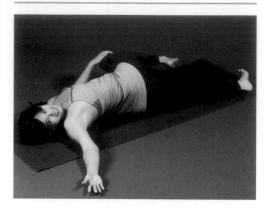

Lie down on your back. Slightly arch your lower back to settle into your body's natural lumbar curve. Pull your right knee into your chest, keeping the slight arch in your spine. Shift your hips toward the right side of your mat as you cross your right knee over your body and lower it toward the floor on your left side. Use a block under your knee for support if it's hovering off the floor. Take your hand to your lower back and feel for a lift in the muscles around your spine. See if you can get the ridge of muscles around your spine to activate. Extend your right arm out and look to the right. Stay here for 10 breaths.

Roll back to center. Make sure you have a gap between your lower back and floor again; you should be able to slide your hand all the way underneath your lower back. Pull your left knee into your chest. Shift your hips toward the left side of your mat. Lower your left knee to the right, supporting it with a block if needed. Feel for the lift in the muscles around your spine again. Extend your left arm out and look to the left. Stay here for 10 breaths.

RECLINED PIGEON STRETCH

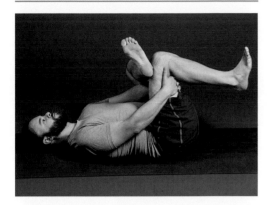

Lie on your back. Walk your feet up to your hips. Cross your right ankle over your left knee, keeping your feet flexed. Reach your right hand between your legs, take your left hand around your left thigh, and interlace your fingers to pull your left leg in toward your chest. An alternative is to move to the wall and prop your left foot up against the wall for the hip stretch. Relax and stay here for 10 to 15 breaths.

Release your hands and place your feet on the floor. Cross your left ankle over your right knee. Reach your left hand between your legs and your right hand around your right thigh, interlace your fingers, and pull your right leg in toward your chest. Flex your feet. Stay for 10 to 15 breaths.

FISH WITH A BOLSTER

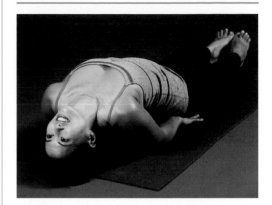

Set up a bolster on the floor lengthwise, or line up a couple of cushions that support your lower back and shoulders. Sit down with the bolster behind you and then lie back across it. If you have neck pain, support your head with a block or additional cushions.

As an alternative to a bolster, from a seated position with your legs straight, slide your fingertips underneath your sit bones. Lower back onto your elbows, keeping your shoulders off the floor. Press into your hands and lift your chest to the ceiling.

Adjust your lower back into a more pronounced curve, tilting your hips forward and down toward the floor. Soften across your chest. Stay here for 10 to 15 breaths.

SHOULDER STRETCH

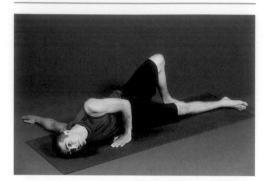

Lie down on your belly. Extend your right arm out at approximately a 90-degree angle on the floor; aim to have your right hand slightly forward of your shoulder on the floor. Pick up your left foot, roll onto your right hip, and bring your foot to the floor behind you. It may be easy to get your foot to the floor; if not, place it down wherever you can while staying in the stretch. Once you're deep into the shoulder stretch, relax for 10 breaths.

For the other side, extend your left arm to approximately a 90-degree angle on the floor; aim to have your left hand slightly forward of your shoulder on the floor. Pick up your right foot, roll onto your left hip, and bring your foot to the floor behind you. Relax for 10 breaths.

HALFWAY LIFT

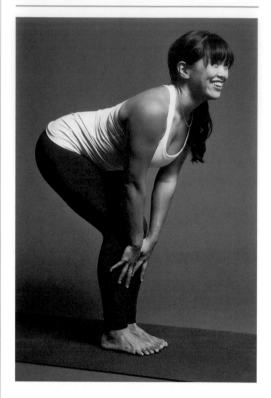

Essentially a hip hinge, the halfway lift challenges you to engage your core, activate your hamstrings, and strengthen your lower back. Stand with your feet together, big toes touching. Connect the four corners of your feet to the floor. Bend at the hips and place your hands on your thighs. Soften your knees and squeeze your shins toward each other. Extend your chest parallel to the floor. Lift your tailbone toward the sky, grounding down into your heels. Hug your shoulder blades onto your spine to stretch your chest. Extend your neck in line with your spine. Stay for 10 rounds of breath.

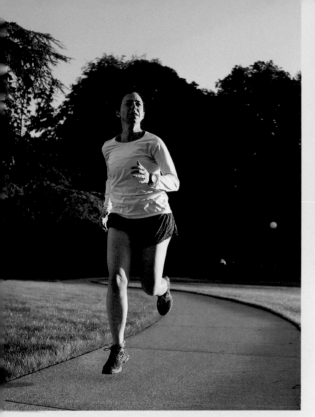

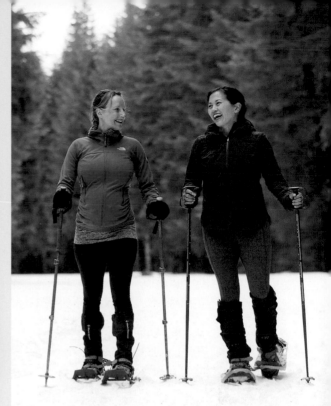

the next
12 months

When my fitness column ended, I wondered if I would try new things without a weekly deadline—a huge motivator for a writer. Would I do the research to find new activities? Would I prioritize the time it takes to get around town to try those classes?

Turns out the answer was no.

I missed trying new classes—a lot. But I did not miss juggling my schedule to fit the one time a class was being offered, nor did I miss fighting traffic to go to a class across the city during rush hour, at least not every week.

So after the end of the column, I took a break. I did my regular movement practices of walking, yoga, and Olympic weightlifting, and I contemplated what was next. I knew I wanted a solution that addressed my biggest lament about the column: I tried new activities all the time but rarely followed through for a second class. I also wanted a solution

that included dance, which I had fallen in love with during the column. I wanted to dance! I missed it, even.

I am a good mimic and not a particularly talented dancer. But over time, I gave up worrying if I was any good, because the truth is, at the beginning you never are. But dance classes plastered a smile across my face. The combination of engaging movement that used my whole body and the mental challenge of following choreography (my favorite type of dance class) was missing from my post-column life. Without the column, dance might disappear.

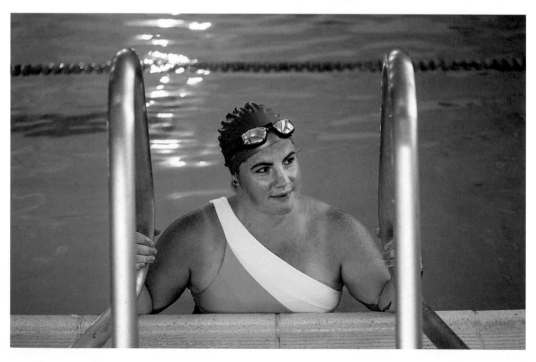

So I looked for a dance class that included the final piece of the puzzle—a location close to home. I picked tap. Part of it was practical—I live near a nonprofit I admire, Northwest Tap Connection, which is dedicated to uplifting underserved communities through dance. Part of it was tap dance. I have tap shoes left over from a short stint in tap in college, and I loved the pizzazz of the dance form and the satisfying sound of shoes tapping in sync. I was in.

The adult tap class ran once a week. As soon as I arrived for class, I realized I had chosen an inopportune time to join, at least from my perspective. The class was preparing for its biannual studio showcase performance, two months out. Not only did the idea of performing sound awful, but it also meant our teacher was pushing the upper end of technical difficulty with the choreography.

The first week, I was basically lost in the steps to our song, "Doesn't Really Matter" by Janet Jackson. My 21-year-old teacher, Rachel, who had grown up taking tap, modern, and hip-hop dance at the studio, patiently broke down the steps to our song for the class over and over again. But I couldn't make my right foot shuffle in time, no matter how hard I tried. When the steps were slow, I had a chance of hitting the choreography. As soon as Rachel sped it up and put on the music, the fast tap pattern was over before I knew it.

I wanted to give up.

Yup, me, the one who has been encouraging you through every page of this book to try something new and stick with it. I didn't want to go back. I wanted to skip tap in favor of weightlifting, where I knew what to do. I didn't want to face up to how much technique

I would have to learn to keep up with other students who had taken tap as kids. I wanted to do anything except embarrass myself in class, again. But I knew the only way to get better was to go back. I gave myself a pep talk and returned the next week.

The second class was marginally better; muscle memory, thank goodness, helped me catch a couple more steps than the week before. I hit maybe 30 percent of the steps, but it was an improvement. It was enough for me to say, "Fine. I'll go back." And I went back the next week, and the next. I barely managed to hang on to the steps we learned and pick up the new ones Rachel added each week.

Soon, class discussion turned to outfits for the upcoming studio showcase. Dancers voted on whether we should wear sparkly tops. I pretended not to pay attention. I wondered if I should perform, if they wanted me to join, even as people asked me if I would be dancing. I was not taking tap class to dance on a stage, I told myself. I dance for me.

But the class was gathering momentum. People recorded Rachel doing the dance and practiced steps at home. Rachel added more choreography. The week of the show, a couple of dancers showed up with sparkly tops to make sure everyone wore a different color.

Decision time. It was now or never. For better or worse, my schedule was clear to spend a full Saturday at a local high school auditorium for two performances. Something out there was telling me to perform.

But I wanted to bail on the performance *so badly*. I wanted to sit at home, without a sparkly top, and without the pressure of performing on a stage in a dance I had just learned. I also knew by this point that if I did sit at home, I would be so mad at myself. For

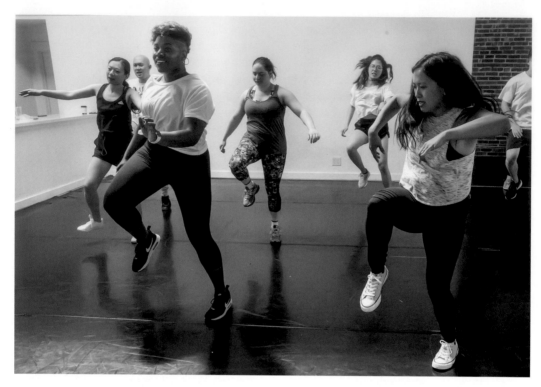

not being brave in a scary situation. For not doing something that terrified me. For not forging a deeper connection to a community I had just joined.

So I got a navy sequin top. I curled my hair. I put on makeup. I spent the entire day with my fellow dancers, hanging out backstage with adults wrapped in bold patterns for African dance and kids wearing butterfly wings for toddler tap. I snuck out to the audience to watch parts of the show and was so moved watching the gifted teenage and child dancers perform that I cried, multiple times.

I did the full tap routine, twice. I smiled, lights bright on my face. I flubbed steps. I hit steps. I was so proud of myself.

By participating in the performance, by continuing to push myself in a class I'd wanted to drop, I had found a new community—and another side of myself.

So—now that your year is up, now that you've tried more activities than you've maybe ever tried in your life, what do you do next? What do you do with what you've learned, with all this information you've gathered about your body, its strength, and its ability to move? What do you do with what you've learned about what movement does for you?

It's time to commit. It's time to take it to the next level. It's time to see what's possible when you apply everything you've absorbed.

You pick one activity. You join a community. You get to know people.

You keep going, even when you don't feel like doing an activity one day. You take a class or you make time on weekends to get better at your new activity. You ski through the whole winter. You swing dance even when you stumble over your partner's feet. You go roller skating, and you learn to derby stop.

You pick your favorites, and you keep doing them. You get better. You do them over and over.

You see what's possible after one year—12 months—of trying new things. You apply what you learned. You show yourself how much you can grow.

HOW TO MAKE THE MOST OF YOUR NEW MOVEMENT LIFE

You did it. You moved for 12 months straight.

Dang. That is huge. First, give yourself a pat on the back. It's a huge accomplishment to commit to move more, no matter whether you tried one activity or got in all 24. (However many you did, please find me and tell me so I can celebrate you, too!)

Second, take a look back. Go read your original Movement Assessment. See what has changed since you first opened this book and decided to transform how much you move. Look back at what you hoped to accomplish and how you felt about yourself when you started. Read over your journal entries throughout the year. Reflect on what has shifted and what you've discovered about yourself and your body in one year: 12 months; 52 weeks; 365 days.

Finally, now that you've cemented all these habits and new patterns over the past year, it's time to go to the next level. It's time to dive deeper and commit to yourself in a new way by taking on just one thing you loved and seeing it through.

You have proven to yourself you can learn to do new things. Now it's time to rise to the next level, mastering skills in a dance class or pushing yourself to a 20-mile walk. It's time to learn techniques that escaped you in the intro class. It's time to see what your body is capable of when you go all in.

This year has been all about priming yourself to go to the next level. I can't wait to see what you do next.

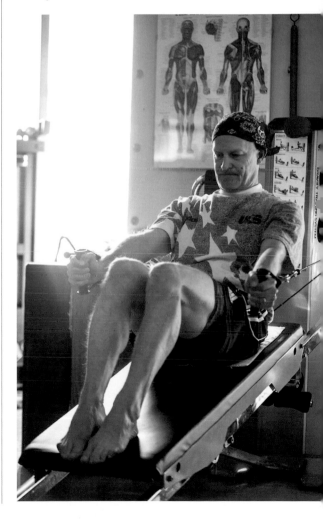

DISCOVERY

What were your goals when you started this movement journey? What intention did you set?

Are you moving more than you did when you started? What have you added in since you started this yearlong movement journey?

What have you learned about your body over the past year? What have you learned about your capacity to learn new things in relation to your body?

What surprised you the most about this year?

When did you have the most fun? Was it learning a new activity, a specific activity itself, or the time when you started to feel confident or comfortable in a new movement?

What can you appreciate about what you did this past year on this movement adventure? Did you experience a shift in physical strength or energy?

What was your favorite activity? What commitment can you make to keep doing this activity for the next 12 months?

JOURNAL

Use these pages to track your progress over the next 12 months, make note of what you love and what you learned, and brainstorm ideas for other activities to try once you are through the year!

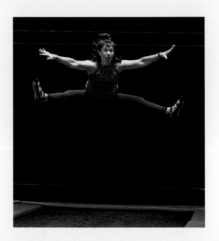

JOURNAL

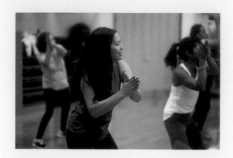

JOURNAL

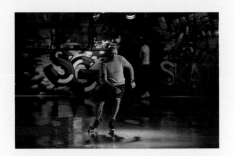

JOURNAL

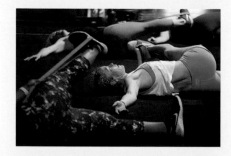

JOURNAL

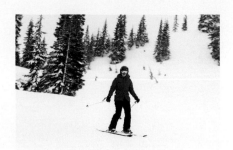

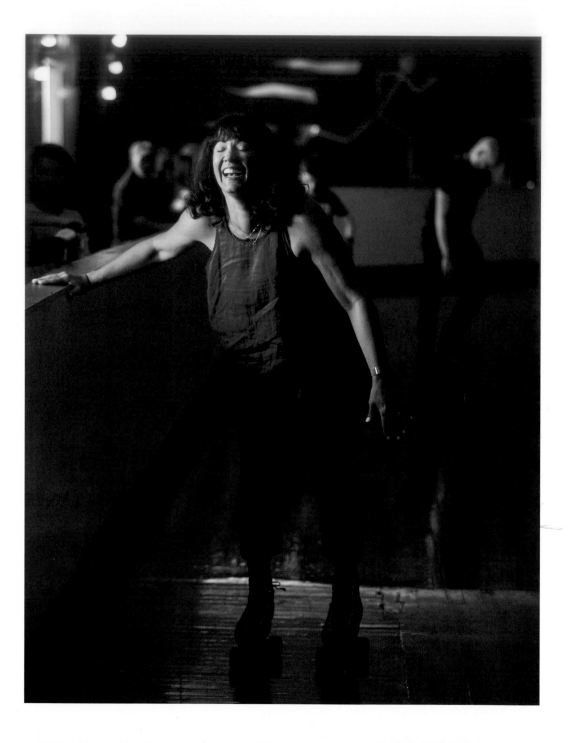

acknowledgments

The credit for this book starts with my earliest movement teachers: my childhood ice skating coach, Yvonne, and my tennis coaches. My yoga teachers taught me to understand my body and myself, guiding me to see how big a life I could lead. Thank you to every movement teacher I ever took a class from for Fit for Life. Thank you, Katy Bowman, for opening my eyes up to a new way of movement and sharing what you do with such grace and joy.

The anchor of my movement community is Rocket Community Fitness in Seattle. Brady and Alyssa, thank you for welcoming me as a new member, for watching my highs and lows in nutrition challenges, for encouraging me to learn Olympic weightlifting, for supporting photo shoots, for gathering the best damn group of humans I know, for making sure I always have a movement home. Thank you to my yoga communities, especially Be Luminous Yoga, for launching me on this movement pathway, keeping me grounded, and always supporting my dreams.

Thank you to *The Seattle Times*, specifically former editors Kathy Andrisevic and Kathy Triesch, for seeing the promise in me and in Fit for Life. Thank you to Bill Reader for taking me all the way across the finish line!

To editors Kate Rogers, Linda Gunnarson, Janet Kimball, Ali Shaw, and the rest of the Mountaineers Books team, thank you for your dedication and diligence to making this book sing. Erika Schultz, I love that you love a crazy project as much as I do! You carry off photo shoots and create stunning images with such talent and good humor.

Thank you to my star fitness models, folks who loaned their time and community for such beautiful images—Courtney McGrue; Chelle Swierz; Clare, Mark, and Ben Megathlin; Natalie Wieder; Christine Bachman; Sarah Greene; Rafe Kelley of Evolve Move Play; Jenny Gawf; Hallie Kuperman of Century Ballroom; Velocity Dance Center; Michael O'Neal; Dana Belkholm of Mind and Body Pilates; Kim Kubota; Max Genereaux; Jen Mulholland; Coach Kim Nguyen and Pacific Muay Thai; Master Yijiao Hong; Southgate Roller Rink; Defy Seattle; Austin Carrillo; Tina Templeman; Brian Charlton; Taylor Moravec; and Genevieve Alvarez.

I wouldn't reach for giant goals and blessings the way I do without my teachers Susanne Conrad, Dr. Kam and Patty Kettering, and my Lightyear and Geotran communities—thank you for holding me to my highest self, always. Thank you to my mom, Joanna, and my dad, Peter, for giving me the space to be physical and curious my whole life.

I am grateful to be part of a family that loves to move. Paige, Reagan, and Carson, you remind me of what is important every day. And my sweet and energetic Coco, while you may not be able to read these words, please know you are my daily movement inspiration.

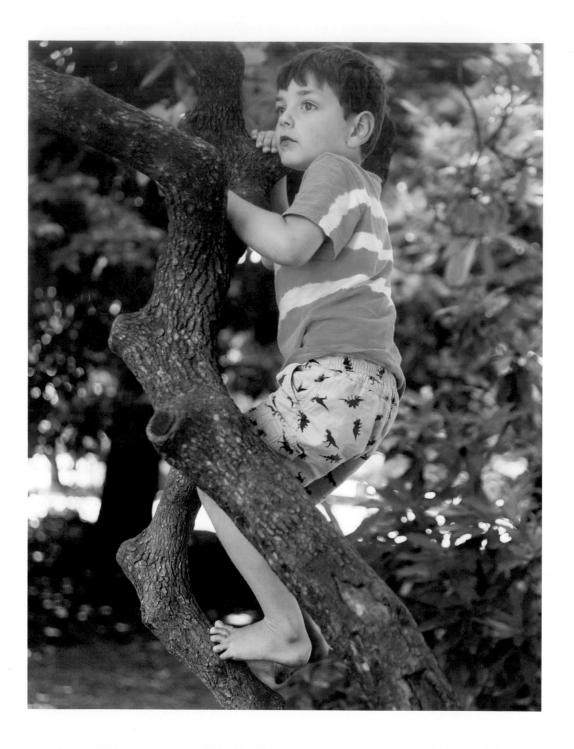

resources

Books

BIKING

Just Ride: A Radically Practical Guide to Riding Your Bike by Grant Petersen (Workman Publishing Company, 2012): Petersen has written an inspirational guide to biking.

Urban Cycling: How to Get to Work, Save Money, and Use Your Bike for City Living, by Madi Carlson (Skipstone, 2015): Here you'll find everything you need to know to make using your bike on a regular basis easy and fun.

Zinn and the Art of Road Bike Maintenance: The World's Best-Selling Bicycle Repair and Maintenance Guide, 5th edition, by Lennard Zinn (VeloPress, 2016): This book shares techniques on maintaining your own bike.

CROSS-FUNCTIONAL FITNESS

Becoming a Supple Leopard: The Ultimate Guide to Resolving Pain, Preventing Injury, and Optimizing Athletic Performance, 2nd edition, by Kelly Starrett and Glen Cordoza (Victory Belt Publishing, 2015): This is an essential book for recovering from intense athletic challenges.

The Power of Community: CrossFit and the Force of Human Connection by Allison Wenglin Belger (Victory Belt Publishing, 2012): Belger is a psychologist who writes about the essential nature of community to improve your life.

HIKING

Look for hiking books that outline trails in your region. Most guides also will include some essentials about gear and how to prepare for the wilderness.

Grandma Gatewood's Walk: The Inspiring Story of the Woman Who Saved the Appalachian Trail by Ben Montgomery (Chicago Review Press, 2016): Read this book about a celebrated female hiker for inspiration about what is possible.

Whole Body Barefoot: Transitioning Well to Minimal Footwear by Katy Bowman (Propriometrics Press, 2015): If you're interested in transitioning to minimal shoes, start with this book.

HIP-HOP DANCE

Beginning Hip-Hop Dance by E. Moncell Durden (Human Kinetics, 2018): Learn both the essentials of dance and the important history of hip-hop culture in the United States.

INDOOR CLIMBING

Better Bouldering, 3rd edition by John Sherman (FalconGuides, 2017): Dig into the bouldering side of things with technique and tricks from John Sherman.

Gym Climbing: Improve Technique, Movement, and Performance, 2nd edition, by Matt Burbach (Mountaineers Books, 2018): Whether you're a novice or advanced gym climber, you'll find what you need in this comprehensive guide.

Mountaineering: The Freedom of the Hills, 9th edition, by The Mountaineers (Mountaineers Books, 2017): This foundational book will walk you through all the essentials needed to start climbing.

The Rock Warrior's Way: Mental Training for Climbers, 2nd edition, by Arno Ilgner (Desiderata Institute, 2006): Dig into the mental side of climbing with this essential climbing book.

KICKBOXING

Complete Kickboxing: The Fighter's Ultimate Guide to Techniques, Concepts, and Strategy for Sparring and Competition by Martina Sprague and Keith Livingston (Turtle Press, 2004): This is a comprehensive guide to kickboxing.

Muay Thai Basics: Introductory Thai Boxing Techniques by Christoph Delp (Blue Snake Books, 2005): Learn both the techniques and the history of Muay Thai boxing.

PILATES

The Pilates Body: The Ultimate At-Home Guide to Strengthening, Lengthening, and Toning Your Body by Brooke Siler (Harmony, 2000): To learn mat Pilates essentials, check out this book by a renowned Pilates teacher.

SKIING

Cross-Country Skiing: Building Skills for Fun and Fitness by Steve Hindman (Mountaineers Books, 2005): Read about the techniques and equipment needed to get out on a Nordic ski adventure.

Ultimate Skiing: Master the Techniques of Great Skiing by Ron LeMaster (Human Kinetics, 2009): This book connects snow, equipment, and movement to give you an introduction to alpine skiing.

SNOWSHOEING

Snow Sense: A Guide to Evaluating Snow Avalanche Hazard, 5th edition, by Jill Fredston and Doug Fesler (Alaska Mountain Safety Center, 2011): If you're headed into the backcountry, read this book to understand the risks and how to keep yourself and others safe.

Snowshoeing: From Novice to Master, 5th edition, by Gene Prater (Mountaineers Books, 2002): This classic guide will get you started on your snowshoe journey.

STAND-UP PADDLEBOARDING

Stand Up Paddling: Flatwater to Surf and Rivers by Rob Casey (Mountaineers Books, 2011): Use this guide to get started or take your paddleboarding to the next level.

Walk on Water: A Guide to Flat Water Stand Up Paddling by Tim Ganley and Vie Binga (Tim Ganley and Vie Binga, 2015): Learn essential paddling skills and how to paddle safely.

SWIMMING

Swimming to Antarctica: Tales of a Long-Distance Swimmer by Lynne Cox (Mariner Books, 2005): While swimming to Antarctica may be a bit aspirational, read for the dedication and inspiration in this memoir.

Total Immersion: The Revolutionary Way to Swim Better, Faster, and Easier by Terry Laughlin (Touchstone, 2004): Master skill drills and improve your form with this guide.

SWING DANCE

Frankie Manning: Ambassador of Lindy Hop by Frankie Manning and Cynthia R. Millman (Temple University Press, 2008): If you want to immerse yourself in the history of Lindy Hop, read the autobiography of one of the innovators.

TABATA

Tabata Workout Handbook: Achieve Maximum Fitness With Over 100 High Intensity Interval Training Workout Plans by Roger Hall (Hatherleigh Press, 2015): Learn more about Tabata and choose from many variations on Tabata workouts in this book.

TAI CHI

The Art of Learning: An Inner Journey to Optimal Performance, 2nd edition, by Josh Waitzkin (Free Press, 2008): While the author earned a world championship title in tai chi, this book is more about his journey about overcoming challenge.

The Complete Book of Tai Chi Chuan: A Comprehensive Guide to the Principles and Practice by Wong Kiew Kit (Tuttle Publishing, 2002): Learn more about the foundational elements and history of tai chi.

TENNIS

Absolute Tennis: The Best and Next Way to Play the Game by Marty Smith (New Chapter Press, 2017): Improve your understanding of tennis technique with this comprehensive book.

TRAIL RUNNING

A Beautiful Work in Progress by Mirna Valerio (Grand Harbor Press, 2017): A memoir details the journey of Valerio, now an ultrarunner, who had a wake-up call at 300 pounds that got her to run.

Good to Go: What the Athlete in All of Us Can Learn from The Strange Science of Recovery by Christie Aschwanden (W. W. Norton & Company, 2019): A resource for runners and athletes alike, this book dives into the science of recovery and cuts through many of the prior claims about it.

TREE CLIMBING

Dynamic Aging: Simple Exercises for Whole-Body Mobility by Katy Bowman (Propriometrics Press, 2017): This book covers how to age well and also includes tips on how Bowman's coauthors started climbing trees in their 70s.

ULTIMATE

Essential Ultimate: Teaching, Coaching, Playing by Michael Baccarini and Tiina Booth (Human Kinetics, 2008): These longtime ultimate teachers guide you through the basics of the sport and how to build a team.

WALKING

The Last Great Walk: The True Story of a 1909 Walk from New York to San Francisco, and Why It Matters Today by Wayne Curtis (Rodale Books, 2014): Learn more about why walking is so essential to being human.

Move Your DNA: Restore Your Health Through Natural Movement by Katy Bowman (Propriometrics Press, 2017): In this book, you'll gain deep insight into why it is so essential to walk and move your body more.

YOGA

The Yoga Bible: The Definitive Guide to Yoga by Christina Brown (Walking Stick Press, 2003): This comprehensive book breaks down the basics for yoga poses taught in Western yoga classes.

Websites

BIKING

Bicycling.com: Read this site for inspiration and practical information.

Map My Ride and Ride with GPS (www.mapmyride.com, www.ridewithgps.com): Look at these sites or download the apps to figure out appropriate routes for biking and track your ride.

CROSS-FUNCTIONAL FITNESS

Breaking Muscle (www.breakingmuscle.com): This site is a comprehensive resource for high-intensity functional fitness and related HIIT movements, with videos and visuals for any of the skill sets you find at gym classes.

PILATES

Blogilates (www.blogilates.com): This site is a go-to for free Pilates videos, including basic mat Pilates workouts and plenty of Pilates inspiration.

STAIR WALKING

Publicstairs.com (www.publicstairs.com): This website is devoted to stair walking around the world. Start here to see if there are stair walking groups in your community or preexisting stair walking maps.

SWIMMING

Your Swim Book (www.yourswimlog.com): This website is a resource for ideas for training once you're swimming. It also has a breakdown of the equipment you need to swim.

SWING DANCE

Lindy Hop Moves (www.lindyhopmoves.com): Come here to learn fundamental and advanced Lindy Hop tricks, with accompanying videos. Trail Running

TRAIL RUNNING

Runner's World (www.runnersworld.com): This site is a hub for running information, training, and resources.

Trail Runner (trailrunnermag.com): Turn here for inspiration and information about training, nutrition, gear, and more.

ZUMBA

Zumba (www.zumba.com): The official website is the best way to find a nearby Zumba class or teacher.

Videos

KICKBOXING

fightTIPS on YouTube: This online channel has beginner videos and tips on technique.

ROLLER SKATING

USA Roller Sports on YouTube: If you want to see good roller skating technique, head to this YouTube channel for beginner tutorials and a lot of inspirational skating.

SWIMMING

GoSwim (www.goswim.tv): If you're looking for videos to master technique, take a look here.

SWING DANCE

Lindy Hop Moves (www.lindyhopmoves.com): Come here to learn fundamental and advanced Lindy Hop tricks, with accompanying videos.

TABATA

20-Minute Tabata-Inspired Workout (www.acefitness.org): If you would like a guided Tabata workout, search for this video on the American Council of Exercise website.

The Fitologists on YouTube: This online channel has videos for people new to Tabata or those looking for a more advanced workout.

TENNIS

Tennis Evolution on YouTube: Watch tips on tennis technique on this online channel.

TRAMPOLINE

Jakub Novotný—Jumping Fitness MT on YouTube: This channel is great for ideas on workouts jumping on a mini-trampoline at home.

ULTIMATE

American Ultimate Academy on YouTube: Check out this channel for numerous video resources that break down how the game works and how to play.

YOGA

Yoga with Adriene on YouTube: This channel has numerous short, simple practices you can follow along from home.

ZUMBA

Zumba on YouTube: The Zumba channel features inspiration, fun music, and some Zumba workouts, too.

about the author

For more than six years, **NICOLE TSONG** wrote the popular Fit for Life column in *The Seattle Times*, published in *Pacific NW Magazine*. Nicole is the author of *Yoga for Hikers* and *Yoga for Climbers* (Mountaineers Books), and has taught yoga for more than a decade, including for three years at the White House Easter Egg Roll.

As a journalist, Nicole lived and worked in Anchorage, Alaska, Washington, D.C., and Walla Walla, Washington, covering topics ranging from the Iditarod Trail Sled Dog Race to a US Senate race. In addition to writing, Nicole currently runs a work/life balance coaching business, supporting high-achieving women in mastering radical change.

Raised in Chicago, Nicole was first introduced to the outdoors in high school during a dinosaur dig in Moab, Utah, and her love of hiking and mountains took off during her years as a student at Dartmouth College. After a stint teaching English to college

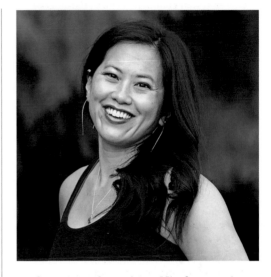

students in Wuhan, China, Nicole moved to the West Coast and has called it home ever since. She now lives in Seattle, where you can find her out in the mountains with her pup, Coco, playing violin, and loving on her houseplants. Reach out at nicoletsong.com.

about the photographer

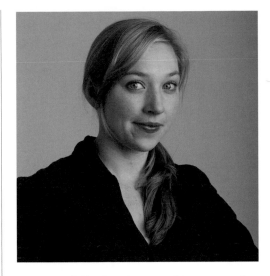

ERIKA SCHULTZ works as a staff photographer for *The Seattle Times*, where she focuses on photo and video storytelling. Schultz teaches photography and video as part-time faculty at the University of Washington's School of Communication.

She has received numerous awards including honors from the 2019 Best of Photojournalism's Online Video, Storytelling and Innovation (with *The Seattle Times* video department) and a 2017 award of excellence for Newspaper Photographer of the Year from Pictures of the Year International. Schultz's work also has been recognized by the Casey Medals for Meritorious Journalism, National Edward R. Murrow Awards, the Alexia Foundation, and the Society of Professional Journalists, among others. She also was part of *The Seattle Times'* 2010 Pulitzer Prize winning team for Breaking News Reporting.

She serves on the Western Washington Board of the Society of Professional Journalists and as a former Artworks Projects Emerging Lens Mentor. Schultz is co-founder of NW Photojournalism and a member of *The Seattle Times* Diversity and Inclusion Task Force.

In her free time, Schultz enjoys running, biking, snowboarding, gardening and learning Spanish. She loves exploring red rocks and slot canyons in the Southwest, retracing her childhood camping spots in Wyoming's Absaroka mountains and hiking on Washington's Olympic Peninsula.

SKIPSTONE is an imprint of independent, nonprofit publisher Mountaineers Books. It features thematically related titles that promote a deeper connection to our natural world through sustainable practice and backyard activism. Our readers live smart, play well, and typically engage with the community around them. Skipstone guides explore healthy lifestyles and how an outdoor life relates to the well-being of our planet, as well as of our own neighborhoods. Sustainable foods and gardens; healthful living; realistic and doable conservation at home; modern aspirations for community—Skipstone tries to address such topics in ways that emphasize active living, local and grassroots practices, and a small footprint.

Our hope is that Skipstone books will inspire you to effect change without losing your sense of humor, to celebrate the freedom and generosity of a life outdoors, and to move forward with gentle leaps or breathtaking bounds.

All of our publications, as part of our 501(c)(3) nonprofit program, are made possible through the generosity of donors and through sales of 700 titles on outdoor recreation, sustainable lifestyle, and conservation. To donate, purchase books, or learn more, visit us online:

skipstonebooks.org
mountaineersbooks.org

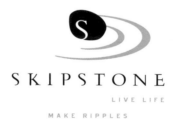

SKIPSTONE
LIVE LIFE
MAKE RIPPLES

YOU MAY ALSO ENJOY:

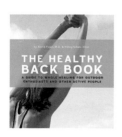 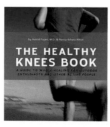 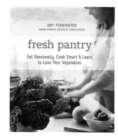 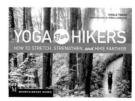